THE LAST DIET

WHERE NUTRITION FAILS.

By

WILLIAM CROWELL

ISBN: 1-4140-2823-7 (e-book)
ISBN: 1-4140-2822-9 (Paperback)

Library of Congress Control Number: 2003097907

This book is printed on acid free paper.

Printed in the United States of America
Bloomington, IN

1stBooks - rev.11/03/03

About the Book

The information in this book is the story of my personal odyssey in understanding how we are affected by food, and how I came discover a way of thinking about food that may be helpful to others. It should not be used as a substitute for consultation with a licensed medical practitioner. You should talk with your physician before initiating any substantial change in your diet.

Table of Contents

Foreword

This book was many years in the writing and more years in the publishing, as it presents a new idea and doesn't fit the niches that various publishers have defined for themselves. It is also not written by a medical professional, but by a layman who found answers to health problems that the medical profession had no solution for. At this point the author, my husband, is well into middle age, still slender and free of heart disease, high cholesterol, diabetes, and many other problems that plague most people our age. He is also in this relatively healthy state without the aid of medications.

The way of thinking about food that he presents is novel, and for an individual to implement it in practice will require some investigation into one's ancestry and the eating

habits of ones ancestors. The effort can be well
worth it.

Sharon Crowell-Davis, 2003

Preface

What's for dinner? Is dinner 'junk' food on the run? Do you just eat something and pop a supplement or do you consider fiber, folic acid, vitamin C, beta carotene, vitamin E, zinc, etc. If you don't take supplements does your daily diet have the Recommended Daily Allowance? What about a vegetarian diet, antioxidants, low fat foods, low cholesterol foods, whole grains, natural foods, organically grown vegetables, etc. Do you think you have problems with natural toxins, food allergies, or food intolerances? Confused?

Today with all the information, scientific studies, medical conclusions, and research, the average person is left with the idea that all this is just cocktail trivia to be taken with a glass of wine which research says is good for you in moderation. There are so many things to consider in diet that even researchers can become confused as to what is important. There is disagreement on many points. Where does all this end?

There is just too much information and too many facts to understand what the best diet to follow is. Order and organization, when applied to all these dietary facts leads to a diet that is far different from what many modern researchers say is best.

When I was in high school one of the books I came across was <u>Silent Spring</u> by Rachel Carson. This book didn't stun my mind the way it had spurred ecological thinking in the general population. At that time I understood it in an entirely different light. The ideas it presented interested me more and more. Humans were using technologies or man made toxins indiscriminately without understanding natural food chains or how the web of life was interconnected as a whole. Bit by bit, I learned about working ecosystems and how we are interdependent upon other life on this planet.

Little did I suspect that it would lead to this book about how humans have ignored ecology in pursuit of a perfect diet. Only a few suspect that this ignorance of the ecology of human diet leads to millions of dollars of wasted medicine.

x

I have an idea that one day my book will inspire someone. One girl who read James Herriot's books became a veterinarian and helped tremendously on this book. Someone may walk up to me and say that my book inspired them.

This book is for the women in science who make a difference. Women like Dr. Rachel Carson, Dr.Dian Fosey, Dr Doris Rapp and Dr. Sharon Crowell-Davis.

13 March 1985 wpcd

Chapter 1

OVERVIEW

Using nutrition as a foundation for human diet and dietary research is like trying to solve a puzzle with only half the pieces. Nutrition is only part of the complex picture of human dietary ecology.

As individuals, we are woven into a web of life so intricate that we are only now beginning to understand how it works. As part of that web we need to understand how tightly we are bound to it. Our physiology, especially our immune physiology, can show how intricately we are connected to the food chain of that web. In other words, our individual physiology, not a collection of generalized facts on nutrients, should dictate the best diet to follow.

Finding how our physiology is connected to ecology is difficult, but by using ecology in human and animal dietary research we may solve some of the most challenging health and medical problems that are plaguing civilization today.

Reading this book will open your eyes to this ecological approach to diet. It is not really difficult for any scientist or non-scientist to understand. You will understand why medical definitions of food allergies and intolerances are inadequate and you will understand why many of the books now written on diet are not really helpful.

The idea in this book is really quite simple. Humans living in a specific local ecology for thousands of years adapted in many ways to the foods available in that locale. Their digestive physiology adapted to the local available foods, as did their immune physiology. Each individual adapted to specific forms of vitamin and mineral compounds from foods in their limited ancestral ecology. The best way for an individual to get these nutrients is to eat a diet as close as possible to the foods their specific ancestors ate. This does not mean the cave men diet. It means the diet that an individual's ancestors lived on for the last few thousand years until just three or four hundred years ago. After thousands of years of human adaptation to specific local ecologies the world and these local ecologies changed almost overnight in evolutionary time.

After Columbus and the age of discovery, people with specific physiological adaptations strayed to different ecologies all over the world. They transplanted their local food crops and animal stocks to distant continents all over the planet, totally changing the local ecology in many areas. This happened long before the beginning of modern scientific investigation.

These immigrant people started adapting to this new local ecology and foods that were available or brought in from all over the world. Interracial and interregional marriages produced all kinds of differences in humans. This has created an extremely complex ecological situation.

The problem is that the physiology in many of these immigrants is still in the process of adapting to this massive but equally swift change in the human diet. Those that left their native ecology have to adapt and are still adapting to this global agricultural ecology. This process of adaptation or, in some cases, failure to adapt, is the cause of many food and dietary problems. The recognition of these problems and solving them is the theme of this book.

Nutrients are tangible molecules that are relatively easy to single out for scientific study, but nutrition is a generalized collection of specific facts that even in total do not describe all dietary parameters. Shifting dietary studies to an ecological point of view introduces a manifold complexity, but this view will be a more complete view of human diet.

Over the last couple of decades, the subject of food allergies and intolerances has provoked much debate. The debate over yeast problems, toxins, and diseases related to the intake of foods, such as arthritis, schizophrenia, or multiple sclerosis is much contested. Indeed, so much debate and disagreement in any scientific field indicates a lack of order. If we used ecological order as a basis for food problems these debates would subside into a clearer understanding of how diet affects the human body.

Anyone with multiple allergies to foods such as milk, whole grains, citrus fruits, and the nightshade family will find it difficult if not impossible to have a "nutritionally balanced" diet. Food allergies are the failings of almost every single diet yet devised. If you are allergic to multiple kinds of grains, then most commonly recommended diets fail. The vegetarian diet, for instance, requires grains as a necessary component to supply protein.

The idea is simple enough. Humans are a product of their ancestral ecology. Every single aspect of human physiology is 'shaped' by adaptation to a specific ecology. The digestion and assimilation of food is a major part of this process. Our physiology, from digestive and immune to fat storage is adapted or adapting to the food available. This adaptation takes many ecological twists and turns, so to speak, because of factors such as marriages between people from different parts of the world. Food allergies and food intolerances derive from an individual being exposed to foods they have little or no ecological adaptation to.

Chapter 2

A NEW WAY OF THINKING ABOUT DIET

Evidence of the evolutionary aspect of food intolerances and allergies is widespread, but widely ignored. Some doctors that specialize in allergies assert that well over 80% of the population has food allergies, but in the medical profession, food allergies and intolerances are only considered to be a minor problem so long as they don't generate anaphylactic shock. I believe they are far more important to understanding human medicine than even the most seasoned medical allergist can imagine.

If one can add nutrients to the diet, then food allergies are elements to take away. By the process of elimination and nutritional insight I was able to find a set of nutritious foods that caused me no allergy or intolerance problems. After I had only eaten the foods that I'd found I had no allergies or intolerances to for over a year, dozens of beneficial physiological changes happened to me. Some of these changes could be attributed to better nutrition, but there were some, such as improving my dyslexic problem, that had nothing to do with nutrition.

This single set of foods benefited me greatly. Besides having no food allergies, no undue toxins, no intolerances, and a relatively good nutritional balance (although I never counted vitamins), this set of foods caused many beneficial things to happen, such as weight loss, cholesterol reduction, body hair growth (I'd been going bald), and skin wrinkle reduction, along with a multitude of other things important in medicine and science today. I uncovered important aspects of human diet that had little or no scientific research.

No one had really emphasized individual dietary ecology that followed specifically the foods ones ancestry was adapted to. Most dietary ideas are generalized collections of facts that supposedly fit the entire population. However, many individuals find that general recommendations about how to eat aren't working for them. Could this be because the general recommendations are inadequate for their individual case?

Many 'experts' have used positive superlatives about dietary ideas they view as correct, yet few seem to have seen the overall picture. Because of this, many people in the USA are confused creatures of habit who would prefer not to give up the over abundance of problem foods or pay attention to their diet. The medical profession is treating the aftermath of problematic dietary habits because doctors are confused about or do not know the true nature of diet themselves. With traditional ideas of human nutrition commanding and consuming most of the scientific attention, there is little medical attention to other ways of thinking about diet.

Once I had 'discovered' that evolution plays a major factor in human diet I was amazed that someone had not simply stumbled into the idea of using it. A friend commented that I had 'discovered nothing important.' "Everybody knows that," she said. BUT I HAD NOT FOUND ANYONE WHO HAD ACTUALLY USED DIETARY ADAPTATION IN MEDICINE. NO ONE IN DIETARY SCIENCE HAD POINTED OUT HOW NUTRITION WAS A SMALL PART OF A WHOLE AND ITS EXACT RELATIONSHIP TO LIFE SCIENCE.

There had been dozens of ecologists talking about the destruction of habitat and food sources for animals and how some animals had 'adapted.' There were 'mentions' in many of the books on food allergies about how adult humans in some areas may have 'adapted' to milk, especially milk sugars over a couple of thousand years. There was a historic reference about how the shift to wheat and grains in the Middle East may have caused a lot of problems. There were charts that showed that the people who had the most problems with wheat were from areas farthest from the Middle East and the Mediterranean and there were charts showing that people who had the most problems with milk were not from northwestern Europe.

There is a very notable Finnish study on heart disease that suggests Finns were 'not adapted' to a high fat, high cholesterol diet. <u>WHAT</u> <u>FOODS</u> <u>ARE</u> <u>THE</u> <u>FINNS</u> '<u>ADAPTED</u>' <u>TO</u>??? No one seemed to have asked this important question.

It has been found that some people absorb nutrients from some foods better than other people. No one seems to emphasize the issue that every single food we eat has to be adapted to in many different physiological ways and that the best diet for any one individual is a diet that this individual is adapted to. This evolutionary adaptation is hardly mentioned among leading dietary scientists and yet it may cause millions of dollars of medical problems. Is evolution a morally sensitive word even to scientists?

'Nutrition', on the other hand commands attention because it has been heavily researched. Is the idea of 'vitamins' easier to sell or do the vitamin manufacturers pay for more vitamin research? Nutritional study has been so intense that 'nutrition departments' were set up in schools to study the nutritional elements of foods. These schools turn out 'registered dietitians' who write generalized ideas on foods and diets, yet these individuals hardly think about an individual's evolutionary adaptation to foods. They simply count nutrients.

A good example might be a Native American Inuit whose diet consists of a virtually 100% meat diet or animal protein diet. Ancestors of these people, having been living in the same place and eating the same food for thousands of years, adapted their digestive physiology to arctic animals and fish according to simple environmental adaptation.

Would the northern Inuit do better on an omnivorous, 'nutritionally sound' diet prepared by a registered dietitian? Would their system work with a 'nutritionally sound' vegetarian diet? Anyone would know that their bodies would do poorly on the great America junk food diet of burgers, fries or potato chips, pizza and a soft drink or, worse, beer. Would these Native Americans do better on a 'cave man's diet' or would they do better on a diet that their own ancestors ate? What would happen if they moved from Canada to Florida? Would they become overweight and diabetic? I have a friend who fits this pattern exactly. The answers to the above questions are obvious.

What we have today in the United States is an ethnic melting pot. Our ancestors may have come from the eastern Baltic islands, the hills of Transylvania, the South China coast, the Ivory Coast of Africa or the Lakota tribe of North America. It may also be a mix. In each case you or I as an individual are most adapted to the foods native to the local ecological area our ancestry hails from, but we can survive with problems on a diet we are not adapted to.

Most modern dietary personnel push the idea of a 'nutritionally sound' diet of foods that many people are not adapted to or may have only a partial adaptation to without any thought to our ancestral ecology.

The dietary shift from a local ecological diet to a global agricultural diet is a very problematic one for humans. The complexities involved in finding an individual's original adaptations are often many times the complexities of nutrition. Sorting through these complexities may well be worth the effort and much more in many cases. The following text describes how I accomplished this for myself, and how you can do it too.

Chapter 3

HOW IT ALL BEGAN

If you're like many people, you may be allergic to various foods you routinely eat and not realize it. It is true that many people do not display any signs of what are commonly thought to be food allergies, but what you don't know can hurt you. Symptoms for some individuals may come and go, and food allergies can mimic or worsen a variety of problems, including arthritis. Colds that start out as viruses can turn into colds that hang on due to allergies. Understanding food allergies is a key to unlocking what has become a scientific mess. I once thought that I didn't have food allergies.

In fact, I would have sworn that I didn't have food allergies. I couldn't have been more wrong.

This book started in the checkout lane at a grocery store of all places. A midnight tabloid headline read, "YOU MAY HAVE FOOD ALLERGIES." The article described everything from itchy skin, itchy eyes and runny nose, to 'low energy,' stiff joints, headaches and muscle aches. 'OVER HALF THE POPULATION HAVE UNDIAGNOSED OR MISDIAGNOSED FOOD ALLERGIES,' the article said.

I had some of these symptoms. I noticed "FASTING FOR A WEEK WILL RID YOUR BODY OF FOOD ALLERGIES, TOXINS AND INTOLERANCES." Any half wit knows these tabloids are for entertainment purposes only, but they do often have some thought provoking articles between the flying saucers and weird wacky curiosities.

"Is this article for real?" I thought. "I've had all of these symptoms at one time or another, but doesn't everybody?" One thing I have learned is that people with allergies are thought to be hypochondriacs. You don't discuss allergies in polite company.

A month later, after a couple of weeks with a 'cold' I went to an eye, ear, and nose throat specialist. "Yes," he said, after checking for a bacterial infection and strep throat, "You could very well have an allergy. Generally, nasal discharge is clear to slightly cloudy with allergies, as you have. Yellow, green or dark is usually an infection. Red or black is blood. I'll prescribe some medication that might help your problem."

I hated the taste of the medication and the side effect of falling asleep within forty minutes of taking it. (They have much better antihistamines now.) At this point I didn't know if I had one of those tricky house dust problems or a food problem. Maybe it was something I was eating. The medication did seem to work.

I was very familiar with nutrition and diets, having once practiced both vegetarianism and ovolacto vegetarianism, and having worked in a 'natural food' store in college. I had over fifty cookbooks, including the <u>Joy</u> <u>of</u> <u>Cooking</u> by Rombauer and Becker and fifteen books on nutrition, including three by Adelle Davis. I read most of these books and I was a true believer in natural foods. I thought I knew more than the average person about food, but it was what I was about to learn that was far more important. What I had learned was just a background for my experiences.

To me, fasting was missing a couple of meals. I also knew that if I suddenly fasted 'cold turkey' I might get a low blood sugar or caffeine withdrawal headache. In order to get ready to fast, I took several days cutting back and gradually weaning myself, especially from caffeine and simple carbohydrates. Within forty-eight hours of starting the fast I was feeling exceedingly better, and after five days I felt better than I had in years, except for being a little hungry. I was sleeping better, and except for being a little tired in the late afternoon I felt like I had some kind of weight lifted off of me. At this time I just drank distilled water to fill my stomach.

After five days I started feeling confused and 'off balance,' but I could move much more freely and my skin didn't itch and 'crawl' as much as it had before.

If the article was true, I did have food allergies. Gone was the morning stiffness, the morning grogginess, and for some odd reason I didn't feel really 'burned out' tired in the middle of the afternoon, as I so often did. Gone also were the 'night sweats', and I slept better than I had in years.

In the two weeks it took me to get a doctor's appointment I went to the University of Georgia science library and read medical texts and the clinical allergy texts to know about what to expect. When I went back to eating, the wonderful feeling vanished.

I bought every new or used book that was available on food allergies, especially those that were mentioned as references in the library. Theron G. Randolph MD, William G. Cook MD, Doris Rapp MD and other Doctors of Clinical Allergies and Medicine had a lot more to discuss than the midnight tabloids.

I CONSULTED A MEDICAL DOCTOR SPECIALIZING IN ALLERGIES. I want to make this very clear. I SAW A DOCTOR SPECIALIZING IN FOOD PROBLEMS. This specialist in both airborne and food allergies confirmed my suspicions, but I was mildly shaken by the food allergies he found by the skin prick method. The whole idea of food allergy was as confusing as it was interesting. There were hundreds of questions I wanted to ask, but as doctors spend very little time with patients I just got in a few questions that only made me more confused. Even the medical texts and a veterinarian wife did not help the confusion. Nothing really added up. I sensed that something was missing.

I was allergic to cow's milk, which had been the mainstay of my diet via such foods as cheeses and yogurt in the lacto vegetarian diet. The skin pricks also indicated I was allergic to oranges and other citrus products. I had always thought that orange juice was supposed to be good for you! I was severely allergic to green beans, which I ate often, and mildly allergic to tea, which generated no symptoms that I could identify. I drank two to four cups daily.

I was severely allergic to real vanilla, which I later learned caused me almost instant asthma. It was one of those foods that I could touch to the tip of my tongue and my entire throat would swell. Luckily, my throat, when totally swollen from vanilla was large enough in diameter for me to breathe!

The skin prick test showed that I was severely allergic to fresh water trout and oysters. Later, when eating them I found that I got hot flashes, red skin, and itching all over within a few minutes. They caused what is termed an anaphylactic shock to my system. The strange thing was that, compared to the other foods like milk products which I had eaten almost daily, I had had trout maybe four times in my life and I had not had oysters for almost twenty years. Why was I more severely allergic to them than milk?

Most of the foods I was allergic to would have gone totally unnoticed had I not gone to the allergist. Either I had adapted in various ways, such as always demanding one hundred percent cotton clothes for my sensitive skin, or I had simply gotten used to a long bout of upper respiratory problems almost every winter. These bouts were often a serious health problem, but I had never before realized that they were related to allergies. When I stayed off the foods cited in the skin prick test, I did feel better, and didn't feel as 'run down' as before. However, I knew skin prick testing was incomplete, and had problems mentioned in the clinical immunology texts.

As all of my skin prick sensitivities were food allergies, the doctor specializing in food allergies gave me a prescribed two week 'allergy finding' diet plan and explained how to find other foods I was allergic to. He explained that the skin prick method of finding allergies was good for finding certain problems, especially for rhinitis, but it would find 30% or less of my food allergies.

One of the main things it indicated was my allergic status, but there may be false positives and other problems he said. One of the more important things he did not say is that people with blood group 'A' are more likely to have allergies. I had blood type 'A' and several other risk factors for allergies.

I retested each one of these common foods (except trout and oysters) to which I had reacted on the skin prick test in order to get a better understanding of exactly what symptoms they caused and what they individually felt like. Tea was the only one that did nothing. The doctor said that I might possibly have had a false positive like this.

By the end of the third week of eating most of the foods I commonly ate, I found six more food allergies, including whole grain oats, and whole grain rice. I was allergic to sweet potatoes, which I loved, and had problems with some other foods in the allergy finding diet.

I WAS DUMBFOUNDED. THE ABSOLUTE WORST PROBLEM I HAD WAS AN ARTHRITIC STIFFNESS IN MY UPPER BACK AND NECK FROM MOST WHOLE GRAINS! The 'soluble fiber' in oats that was said to reduce cholesterol was the same element that caused me the arthritic problem!

Suddenly, absolutely nothing that anyone wrote about food made any sense. Whole grains were THE 'natural food' and were supposed to be one of the best foods one could eat, but with some of them I got stiff joints every time I ate them. I was the first patient this allergist had had who reported arthritic stiffness from grains, but within weeks he had another.

At this time the major arthritic foundations did not recognize foods as causing any arthritic problem. But there was no question in my mind I had the problem. I fasted, eating only rice three different times and then oats three different times following the allergy text rules to the letter. I couldn't ignore pain and it is hard to tell myself that it is not hurting, although I have seen people that could do exactly that. It was really true I was allergic to these grains, because when I was off them I had no stiffness or pain in my upper back.

Needless to say, this got my attention! I considered myself one of the faithful, ascribing to the whole grain goodness theory. 'An apple a day' would have destroyed me, as I got a similar stiffness in response to eating apples.

Food allergies made mince out of the common knowledge I had about 'natural' foods, vegetarianism, which was dependent on grains for a complete protein balance, and diets in general. After searching the entire University of Georgia library there was not one single diet or dietary idea that fit my allergies.

Wheat products were a different story. I had virtually no problem with some brands of whole wheat flour and yet 'white' flour caused me problems of joint pain. What was going on? At this point I discovered that it helped to check the labels. It seems that during the refining process the major flour milling companies put in ingredients that my immune system reacted to! I was allergic to malted barley, beer etc. I learned the rule that **THE MORE INGREDIENTS THERE ARE IN A FOOD PRODUCT, THE MORE LIKELY IT IS**

THAT YOU WILL REACT TO THAT FOOD PRODUCT. I had to stick to the very basic foods.

I began 'fortifying' my immune system, as the books on nutrition recommended, with vitamins and minerals, when suddenly my immune reactions to foods became worse! The immune system reacts to 'foreign protein' no matter the source. It could be the foreign protein of a pathogen or a food. If you fortify the immune system with vitamins and minerals to act more strongly, then food allergies in my case, become more fierce. No one had told me this would happen either.

FORTIFYING YOUR IMMUNE SYSTEM WAS SUPPOSED TO BE THE GREATEST THING IN THE DIETARY UNIVERSE TO DO TO BE HEALTHY. **IN THIS CASE I WAS BETTER OFF NOT HAVING A NUTRITIOUS DIET, AS I WAS REACTING TO MORE FOODS MORE FIERCELY!**

At this point I discovered that the vitamins I took were giving me asthma! I was allergic to one or more of the ingredients used in the manufacture of the vitamins. Taking these vitamins most winters was possibly why those miserable winter coughs had hung on so long! Luckily it was spring. Doing the 'right thing' nutritionally was TOTALLY WRONG for me.

There were dozens of little things, such as taking vitamins, which turned everything I had read upside down. Food allergies were just as much part of my diet as any other part, such as nutrition. Good nutrition just made my immune system react more fiercely to food allergies, even some foods I had not reacted to before! How backwards can things get!

There were two bits of advice that helped me in this upside down world. "IF THINGS ARE REALLY CONFUSING, WRITE EVERYTHING DOWN IN A FOOD DIARY," the doctor told me. Confusing was not the word. I was totally lost! I not only kept a food diary on my computer but I also wrote every thought and everything I learned worth noting on the subject. The things I wrote down did indeed eventually help me. Eventually, it was the basis for this book as I wrote down the questions I had and the answers as I got them, plus any afterthoughts. More importantly, I made a note of where every diet and everyone writing about diet had failed. They had failed because they hadn't developed a diet or written about the diet that I, as an individual, needed. All the diet books I had read took a "one size fits all" approach.

The second bit of advice came from my wife Sharon. "READ EVERYTHING YOU CAN FIND ABOUT THE SUBJECT AND THIS MAY ANSWER SOME OF YOUR QUESTIONS." I voraciously read everything everyone wrote about diet. I read about immune and digestive physiology and I read about individual foods, their origins, production, and where they grew best. I read and scanned thousands of articles, books, and journals in the University of Georgia library, but no one had written on exactly how food allergies are related to diet. Every diet book either ignored them or 'worked around' them.

It was like an Agatha Christie or Arthur Conan Doyle mystery. Nothing was as it seemed and nothing made real sense. There were too many people saying too much that didn't make sense or fit together. There was too much contradiction and too much confusion even among the 'experts' on the subject of diet and food allergy. There was something very important missing, including the answers to my questions. Everything has to fit together in science, to the point that there is no confusion.

Six weeks later I was standing in the same grocery store line looking back at the rows of food thinking how much difference those six weeks had made. Most of the foods on those rows had ingredients I was allergic to. The surprises kept coming.

Chapter 4

FINDING A SOLUTION

Once I understood what food allergies were, what they felt like in me, and how to find them, I discovered that I had more than even the doctor had described. The number was mounting swiftly, as many as two a week as I continued my diet trials. My reactions to the foods I was allergic to got worse as I got, overall, healthier.

The worst problem I had occurred during the first three months. The start up was extremely confusing because I would often have more than one food that caused the same problem or reaction. It was difficult finding 'safe foods' that did not generate any reactions. I did get the feel for finding my worst food problems, but at times I felt anorexic. As my diet changed from day to day and week to week, it was especially confusing to those around me who cooked.

Using the clinical allergy books as a guideline I set up my food allergy finding diet in as streamlined a system as possible. Generally I started 'testing' or eating a food on Sunday at lunch or supper. I ate the food I was testing two or three times a day over the next few days for up to a week, unless I had definitive symptoms on Monday.

Many of my reactions occurred twenty to twenty-eight hours after I first ate the food, although the worst ones started appearing within seconds after eating the food. If the reaction happened on Monday I could test another food starting as early as Wednesday.

No matter how minor it seemed, I duly wrote down every single detail. Anything and everything that happened, such as my thumbs getting itchy or my hands getting stiff, I would write down. The problem here was that I did not notice everything, or there were 'silent' or 'hidden' reactions as the allergy texts called them.

I learned how to get in contact with myself and notice what was happening to my body. It is similar to meditation and biofeedback. Here I realized that there is a threshold at which people take notice of things. It is like trying to carry on a conversation when there is a lot of background noise. Sometimes when there is a lot of background noise it is difficult to hear what other people are saying. You have to make an effort to hear people speak in such noise. This is the way it was with some of the effects of food allergies.

'Listening' to what was happening to my body was hard at times. Many of the things that were caused by food I had previously thought were 'normal.' If my back got itchy, it was just itchy. I didn't realize most of the 'positive' foods in the skin prick test caused my back to get itchy. So it was a minor detail that hardly bothered me. Itchy, sensitive skin was something that I had always had and was just used to. Some foods caused me such incredibly minor problems that they were not a real bother. This did not mean, however, that I was not allergic to them. I duly noticed all the reactions I could possibly notice. For a long time I never realized that I snore when I eat a serving of corn or popcorn in the evening.

If I rated my worst allergies as ten I would find some reactions that wouldn't count as a one, but then again I might miss a reaction that was as high as three on the scale. I can see people missing reactions as high as six or seven. When I 'fortified' my immune system with vitamins the reactions would go up on this scale for almost every food that I was allergic to. Some reactions, like my cholesterol, fluctuated up and then dropped, but I would have not sensed these without my doctor's tests. There were several 'silent' things such as this that I did not or would not have noticed. When I had identified all the foods I was allergic to and eliminated them from my diet, my cholesterol finally ended up in the 145/155 range.

If I had any doubt about the reaction to a food, or if the test was interrupted, I tested it again. Eventually, I would retest every single food at least three times to make absolutely sure that I had the same reaction to it.

Some reactions, such as my response to pork, were so extremely painful that I did not deliberately test them again for eight years. I 'accidentally' ate pork three more times in testing with the same extremely painful and unpleasant muscle cramps and 'cricks.' I decided to never eat pork again.

I stuck with this testing long after even the most persistent patient would have, simply because I had to find out why all of these wonderful ideas about natural foods and nutrition were wrong for me. I had been taught a lot of things about foods since the first grade, only to have much of that knowledge not fit into this puzzle.

I was indeed secretly 'obsessed' with the idea of finding answers to my questions, because most of what scientists and nutritionists said about foods often did not apply to me. I had to find answers to why everything seemed puzzling and 'backwards' to what was generally believed about foods. After almost six months I had learned a lot of things but I had 'discovered' nothing to really answer my questions. Most of my important questions remained unanswered.

'WHY WAS THIS HAPPENING TO ME?' was the question I wanted answered most.

The list of my food sensitivities had mounted to over three dozen of the more common foods. It also seemed that I was more allergic than I had been before or that my immune system acted more aggressively. I was becoming afraid that I would be 'allergic to everything' as some top allergists described in the clinical allergy texts. I was allergic to virtually every ingredient in my favorite sausage pizza and to the soda with real vanilla which I liked to drink with it! Ice cream and all those fabulous cheeses were out. 'At first you want to cry,' but I knew I had to find answers to all this seeming contradiction.

EUREKA!!!

It was then that I went with Sharon to help her with her horse behavior research. I sat and watched a horse eat grass. Suddenly, the basic question popped into my head and it was then that I realized that I was not getting the whole picture and limiting my questions.

"WHY ISN'T THE HORSE ALLERGIC TO GRASS?" The question was amazingly simple, but the simple answer represented a dramatic shift in how to look at food allergies. Having ancestors that ate grass for thousands of years this horse was probably adapted to it or not allergic to it. With dozens of problematic foods, **WHY NOT FIND FOODS THAT I WASN'T ALLERGIC TO AND NEVER EVER WOULD BE.**

From all the research I had done and all the books I had read I didn't remember anyone, including medical professionals, even remotely mentioning the idea. Most allergy texts flatly stated "There is no such thing as a permanently non-allergenic food." This is from Food Allergy, by Herbert J. Rinkel MD, Theron G. Randolph MD, Michael Zeller MD, published by Charles C. Thomas, 1953 p.61. If this statement were true why wasn't the horse allergic to grass?

Food allergies were screwing up dietary ideas built by thousands of scientists, but none had looked at non allergy foods. Why not use the reverse concept? Instead of a nuisance, food allergies would become a focus point.

I had tested foods with no immediate reaction, but I wasn't sure that I could find foods that caused absolutely no reactions for the rest of my life. The allergy texts were generalizing at this point, and I knew from ecology that they were.

HOW WOULD I KNOW THESE FOODS I WOULD NEVER BE ALLERGIC TO?

Some of the foods I ate produced no reaction at first, but I often became sensitized to them over weeks and months of eating them. Every single allergy text said to 'rotate foods' to prevent this, but that was almost impossible for me, because I was running out of food options and I had to eat 'something' especially after I fortified my immune system to react more strongly to food allergies.

I realized that <u>every</u> <u>single</u> <u>animal</u> on this planet, including humans, had an ecological niche. This natural niche was certainly composed of foods that the animal wasn't allergic to and never would be. This would involve evolutionary adaptation. Over millions of years the panda had evolved a digit especially for dealing with bamboo leaves. It could not possibly be allergic to bamboo. The koala had certainly adapted and was not allergic to the smelly toxic eucalyptus which they feed on year round.

When Sharon was attending Cornell University we lived in the same apartment complex as Dian Fosey. I had talked to her for hours about how mountain gorillas related to their environment and what they ate. During those original conversations, I had never even thought about how human diet related to ecology, except in a very superficial way. Years later, as I thought about everything I had learned about ecology, I realized that there should be foods to which I was not allergic, in theory anyway

As no one had written about how to find foods that a person wasn't allergic to and never would be, I would have to devise my own method of finding foods I was not allergic to. In hindsight, the method I used to find the foods I was tolerant of was actually the hard way. However, no one had even thought of the idea before, and I was still able to find these foods.

With all the nutritional research, I realized that the body needed a relatively balanced set of specific nutrients. Taking a page from nutrient research I selected a single vitamin to deal with. I selected vitamin C, as it was a relatively necessary vitamin, and used the lists of vitamin C foods that were composed by other researchers over the years.

If humans had come this far over the hundreds of millennia needing vitamin C then it had to be supplied by a 'natural' food. The idea was to simply cross my food allergy list with the foods found to be high in vitamin C. I had allergies to over half of the foods high in vitamin C, but there were other reasons to disregard any one of these foods.

For instance, I was allergic to all citrus products, which are well known to have high vitamin C levels. I get stiffness in my fingers, hips, and lower back from the vitamin C rich tomato-pepper-potato family of 'night shade' foods. I also have upper back stiffness with the 'pectin' of apples and pears and other fruits which are good sources of vitamin C. Strawberries had a very short season and yet vitamin C has to be taken in almost daily. I could not imagine anyone eating two cups of parsley a day for vitamin C.

Broccoli was left at the top of the final cross list. I did not appear to be allergic to it in my first tests of a week and it was rich in vitamins and minerals and had a long season in some areas.

I didn't even particularly like it. I had to learn how to buy the best and freshest and to prepare it without condiments or cheese. One of the reasons I didn't like it was that no one had fixed it the way I like to eat it. I liked it fresh and very lightly steamed or just dropped into hot soup. Freezing broccoli incorrectly often broke down the cell walls and made it have mushy unappealing texture.

But broccoli has a negative in that if it is eaten in any quantity it removes iodine from a person's physiology. I also consumed very little iodized salt in my diet. To match broccoli I would have to select a food from the sea. Kelp from the ocean had lots of iodine but the protein would be low. As I needed protein and I had not tried fish, I selected ocean fish.

Because of my extremely severe allergy to trout I was hesitant, but I realized from reading in the texts that there was a difference between fresh and salt water fish. I selected sardines and herring, as these fish were low on the food chain and would not collect and concentrate as many toxins in their fat as tuna or mackerel do. I had extremely painful headaches from coral reef toxins collected by tuna that feed in tropical waters.

As a kid I had eaten these canned fish and loved them. These canned fish with bone in would also supply calcium lost from the milk allergy. I also knew that they had relatively high values of zinc.

Foods that had passed my first round of eating for a week in the allergy testing diet were added. This included sunflower seeds, cauliflower, almonds, carrots, cabbage, green peas, lettuce, and cucumbers, but later I added chicken and turkey. Note that many of these foods were culled from the top of the nutrient charts.

IF ANY FOOD AT ANY TIME GAVE ME ANY PROBLEMS I TOOK IT OFF THIS LIST IMMEDIATELY. Some foods, such as parsnips I had no trouble with, but I could not stand to eat them consistently. I could never figure out how to prepare them to my liking. There were dozens of reasons for selecting or not selecting foods for this list that are too complex to mention. I used mostly nutritional values, the idea of edibility and sometimes 'heresy' (sound nutritional foods were also in this category) about which foods to avoid and which to add, but as always these foods had to be foods that I had no problems with.

Turkey was the exception. I noticed that I could eat it consistently, but I could eat only one serving a day as I would get headaches from it in larger quantities. In large quantities there is a chemical in it that is known to cause headaches in people. I didn't appear to be allergic to it.

At first, I used this diet for allergy testing as all of the foods were 'clear' of reactions. After nine months I started having asthma problems from almonds. My asthma problem with almonds started very strongly with a common cold. There were no symptoms or reactions before the cold. I started having very minor skin reactions to green peas after a gastrointestinal virus. This is the only reaction that abated over the next several years. Why, I don't know.

Pure chocolate didn't seem to give me reactions when I first tried it. When I was in college chocolate consumed with milk often caused me severe headaches. With real vanilla it caused me asthma. For thirteen and a half months I ate three and a half ounces of chocolate twice a week without any problem. Then, when I had a sore throat, problems began. Consumption of chocolate made my hands and hips stiff.

I wasn't certain I had found foods I would never become allergic to, but as always I dropped foods I had any reactions to. I still had in my mind a doctor's statement that a person can become allergic to any and all foods, but I reasoned that an animal's ecological niche is composed of specific foods which the animal wasn't allergic to.

After eating some of these foods consistently for more than a year my immune system still had no reaction to them. I still wasn't certain that I had found foods I was not allergic to and never would be, but I knew that if they caused me no problems after eating them daily for this long then I was getting close.

At this point I wished that there were some kind of verification to assure me that my 'list' was correct. How would I be able to confirm my list?

Suddenly there came a break or, should I say, several fast breaks. It came from talking to people and reading books outside of diet and physiology.

I was looking in a book on Vikings, hoping to find a picture of a Viking boat so I could build my son a bed with this motif. I happened to run upon a section in the book of what the Vikings ate.

THERE IN PRINT WAS A DIET EXTREMELY SIMILAR TO THE DIET I HAD PUT TOGETHER! The Viking ate small fish such as herring. They ate 'sea' cabbages, which are the ancestors of the cabbage, broccoli, and cauliflower family we eat today. They also ate parsnips and carrots. They also ate all manner of berries, birds, bird eggs, and animals found in abundance in the Baltic and North Sea estuaries.

The surprises kept coming. Within hours I was talking to my brother about my find. He had been researching our paternal genealogy in Europe. The name Crowell had been Anglicized from the name Krauel. Two brothers with this name left Rotterdam for America in early 18th century. My brother had found this Krauel name in Finland.

With blond hair, blue eyes and fair skin I knew I had found what I was looking for. I was elated, to say the least. Most of my ancestors came from Viking settled areas or areas controlled by the Vikings. I had found a set of foods that I would never be allergic to.

This is not to say that all my ancestors were Norse. I had ancestors from other cultures and other areas of Europe. These areas of Europe had (note the past tense) completely different ecologies, and I checked out each and every one against my foods. Foods like garbanzo beans, lentils (Mediterranean) and apples (southeastern Europe), and grapes did not fit my pattern. Each food allergy eliminated a specific ecology and the areas where that food grew best. As I had a problem with grape pectins, my French ancestry was not the one I inherited my immune unresponsiveness from!

Medical allergy texts had not even mentioned that there were foods that a person could never be allergic to much less a whole set of them. And this set was found where a specific ancestor had lived for eons of time and adapted to the foods which were found in that local ecology. This ancestor in my case happened to be straight down the paternal lineage.

Having read a variety of medical texts and library articles I knew that I had found an extremely useful bit of information. It stunned me to think that virtually all of my ancestors had survived two hundred and fifty years away from the Scandinavian seas and this specific ecology and these foods, yet my immune physiology recognized them and did not react to them. I had found a solid connection that all of us have to the web of life.

Having read hundreds of articles, periodicals, and books on diet and immune physiology I was amazed that no one had made the connection between human diet and a specific ecology before. There were suggestions to the that effect, such as the fact that some people absorb nutrients from certain specific foods better than other individuals, but the major medical texts and major dietary texts made no mention that individual human physiology was even remotely connected to a specific local ecology and that eating foods outside of this ecology would cause physiological problems. There are some clinical immunologists who do suggest that allergies are foods that an individual is not adapted to, but finding the specific ecological adaptation apparently isn't standard practice.

It was eating this diet consistently over a long period of time that was the key factor. It was the final or last diet that science can find. Having been to over a dozen general practice doctors for undiagnosed food problems convinced me that the medical profession needs to learn HUMAN DIETARY ECOLOGY as a basic. They need baseline studies on medical problems caused by foods.

One thing I did find was a bit of research that suggested immune unresponsiveness (things that your immune system does not respond to) is transmitted paternally in research breed Swiss mice. If this phenomenon holds true for humans then one could simply follow the male lineage through an unchanged name to the 'old country' to find these foods that the immune system does not react to. This is apparently true in my case. It would be too easy, and may not be the case for everyone.

These foods that my immune system does not respond to appear to be inherited in relatively large cohesive units from my paternal side. Was this a 50/50 chance or could these large blocks of immune unresponsiveness be inherited straight through the paternal line. I wish I knew. Note that my food allergies or immune responses to specific foods were inherited from both sides of my family. It is the immune <u>unresponse</u>, or foods which cause me no allergies that come as a block. Note that immune response (allergy) and immune unresponse are exactly opposite.

How easy would it be to find this block of immune unresponsiveness in any one individual? Could the medical profession make use of this large block of immune unresponsiveness to tailor medication and drugs to the individual? Could this diet be useful in other areas such as immune suppressed individuals or AIDS patients?

I looked at the list of my food allergies and realized what I should have realized all along. ONE HUNDRED PERCENT (100%) OF THE PLANT FOODS I HAD PROBLEMS WITH WERE NOT INDIGENOUS OR NATIVE TO WHERE PEOPLE WITH BLONDE HAIR, BLUE EYES AND FAIR SKIN COME FROM (islands of the Baltic area of Scandinavia, to be specific in my case).

The question of 'why was this happening to me?' was answered. I know now why the vegetarian diet did not work for me. If the clinical medical definition of food allergy was changed to point out these ecological facts, I would have had no problems understanding what food allergies were and they would have been easy to find and much easier to deal with from the VERY beginning. Had I been taught this in college I probably never would have had serious allergy problems.

For instance, I was allergic to more than half the foods on the allergy finding diet that the allergist doctor told me to start with. Sweet potato pie was one of my favorite foods and sweet potatoes were on the allergy finding diet. It was a food from the Caribbean Islands and I, as a Nordic individual, was allergic to it. If the doctor could have handed me a diet consistent with my features and explained a little bit of the ecology of diet I would have found my answers much sooner.

One thing I noticed is that the longer my ancestors had eaten a food not native to Scandinavia the less likely I it was that I would have problems with it. The minor problems with some foods not native to Scandinavia were with foods my grand parents and old timers remember their parents and grand parents eating. Foods grown or cultivated during the time my ancestors were in Middle Tennessee fall into this group. Corn, some beans, 'field' peas, some squashes, hickory nuts and walnuts. It was simple enough to go back and read what people in Middle Tennessee ate before the Civil War. It did not surprise me about the nuts and acorns in 'hard times.'

Another thing I noticed was that foods run in family groups and the protein, carbohydrates, and fats in those foods are similar. The cabbage or cruciferae family includes cabbage, sea cabbage, broccoli, cauliflower, mustard, horseradish, and kale. The sunflower or compositae family has Jerusalem artichoke, sunflower seeds, lettuce, and lettuce seeds.

Using human dietary ecology in research, scientists could know if a food or foods are the cause of, or contribute to diseases as diabetes, multiple sclerosis, and cancers. What would this diet do for immune suppressed individuals? Thousands of research papers could be written in this area alone.

For instance, in modern times Native Americans of the Northern plains have one of the highest diabetic rates in the USA. Their ancestors did not eat grains as a major part of their diet. Natives of the American Southwest ate corn, but did not eat wheat. Their diabetic rate is lower. Some allergists think alcohol addiction is related to allergies of the ingredients from which the alcohol is made. As I have pointed out, food allergies are simply foods one's ancestors didn't eat in abundance.

I learned in my middle school days where most of the foods I was allergic to came from. Chocolate and vanilla were originally from Mexico. Tomatoes, green and chili peppers, were originally from Central America, while potatoes were from Peru. Cloves, ginger, and some pickling spices were from the Far Eastern tropical spice islands. Oranges and citrus came from the South China-Thailand area. Tea was from the Assam region of India while coffee was from Ethiopia. Tea, which at first seemed like a false positive because I had no symptoms, was actually an allergy with no overt symptoms. Most grains I had arthritis from were not introduced into Northern Europe until late from the Middle East or Southeast Asia or Africa.

Following an ecology guideline makes food tolerances, food allergies, food intolerances, and toxins associated with foods predictable. I will describe this later. This is something that clinical food allergists do not now do. I called the local clinical allergy specialist about my ideas. When we got to the part about the surname, but long before I could explain everything to put it all together he threw up red flags. "Genealogy is unreliable and meaningless in scientific research. End of conversation… I don't want to hear any more, period and that is final. Good-bye".

I can see this doctor's point of view. He had just left one of the foremost food allergy clinics in the nation where he was an intern. He was board certified in all areas of immunology including rheumatology. Do you think that with all this medical training he is going to listen to a patient who thinks he knows a few things about food allergies that are not in the books! The problem is that he did not know evolution and ecology very well and he did not realize food allergies followed or might follow a very specific ecological order. I called several other doctors and they were just to busy with their practice to get their mind into human dietary ecology.

Nutrition becomes a non point, so to speak. The foods in one's ancestral ecology will have all the necessary nutrients and they will be better absorbed and/or far better utilized. Tests have shown that some people absorb certain nutrients from specific foods better than others. There might also be nutrients that nutritionists do not now recognize. Nutritionists could learn exactly how much of which nutrients an individual actually needs.

The current medical definition of food allergies is incomplete and therefore confusing.

If food allergies were defined in ecological terms there would be more people with food allergies and intolerances than the medical community now recognizes.

Within weeks I would have to test these ideas on my son, yet it wasn't only my son that would help me discover how extremely important this diet based on evolution and ecology really was.

After this 'discovery' I made these ancestral foods the major part of my diet and tried to find other foods from my discovery of the area of the world my ancestry hailed from. Some more than incredible things happened along the way. Many of the things that happened to me were and are problems which doctors now use chemicals and drugs to treat patients for. Even I didn't understand at first how incredible this ecological set of foods really was.

Chapter 5

SOME IMPLICATIONS

Until the time of the great explorers such as Columbus, most people lived within a hundred miles of where their ancestors had lived for untold millennia. There were a few exceptions, such as armies, but these people were few in number compared to the general population.

Basically, the human population developed and adapted to local conditions of climate, pathogens, and foods readily available in the local ecology. Some adaptations were short term and some last as long as there is a survivor of that genetic line. Some of these adaptations may take several millennia while some may take as little as five or six generations.

The digestive and immune physiology also may have adapted to these local foods in subtle and often undescribed ways. For example, Guatemalan Native Americans whose ancestors lived on corn and beans can assimilate a native corn and bean diet far better than an Eskimo whose ancestors have lived on a diet consisting of 100% arctic animals and fish. This is not to say that a Guatemalan Native American could not survive on arctic animals and fish or vice versa, but that if the switch is long enough, subtle or even overt problems with food allergies and food intolerances will eventually show up in one form or another. The immune system of the Eskimo who has not 'experienced' corn will 'view' its protein as foreign and develop an allergy to it. Or the Eskimo could develop diabetes, having not dealt with the starches from corn and beans. But conversely the Guatemalan may or may not develop problems with the arctic animals and arctic fish.

One problem today is that we have a melting pot, or mixed heritage society that doctors have to treat. I will admit that I had a relatively easy time finding my heritage, which was already researched by others in my family. Most of my family can be traced as far back as seven to eight generations on all sides and/or to a specific area of Northern and Western Europe.

This does not negate the idea. It does make some people have to work harder to find their ideal diet.

I had a girlfriend with allergy and intolerance problems whose mother was French/Vietnamese and whose father was Irish/Apache Native American. Her Vietnamese ancestry was part Chinese and her Irish ancestry was part Scottish.

Could the day come when we punch information into a computer such as such as a Greek nose, genealogy, blood type, and some other features such as a Human Leucocyte Antigen (HLA) profile and specific protein factors to come out with a near perfect diet?

We also have a Global Agricultural Ecology to deal with. An individual's physiology has to deal with every aspect of the dietary change from their ancestral ecology. Potato toxins from the green skins and potato eyes will often abort a fetus in European women while the native women of Peru whose ancestors had the potato for a staple have little or no problems from it.

Ochratoxin from a fungus which grows on maize and beans causes kidney disease along the Danube in Yugoslavia and Bulgaria. You will note that maize and many beans are native to the Americas and not to the Danube region. This dietary switch world wide may cause untold disease problems not really 'seen' by doctors and scientists for what they really are. Every individual has to adapt to every aspect of their dietary ecology. This ecology also includes the fungi, bacteria and other minute organisms that grow on food.

Research suggests that if a person with kidney disease cuts back on protein then the kidneys will not deteriorate as swiftly. This is another generalization. What is the consequence of a person eating specific proteins that they are or are not adapted to? Can the person eat specific protein foods as long as they follow adaptive patterns? This is another area that needs research.

Humans are also adapting to alcohol, tobacco, and drugs. Each time a fetus lives or is spontaneously aborted, each time an infant dies of asthma or other problems related to these vices, or survives, there is evolutionary adaptation.

I learned which foods my ancestors had available in America that were partially and/or mostly adapted to. It becomes simple when you realize that it takes several or many generations to adapt to a set of foods. The longer your ancestors have been eating a food the more you are likely to be adapted to it and the fewer problems you will have with it.

It is difficult to imagine dozens of these adaptations going on at once along with pathogenic organisms, etc. challenging the entire human system. It may help explain why the United States has a higher infant mortality than a more homogeneous country such as Sweden. Indeed, human diet may be the best example of displaced ecology and/or human evolution yet.

Chapter 6

MINOR ISSUES AND MAJOR ISSUES

It sounds terribly mundane that all this started from a reading a 'midnight tabloid' while standing in the check out line at a grocery store. The idea might wind up as a sensation in these tabloids yet. I don't want to give anyone the idea that my food problems were really a problem. I hardly noticed that I had food allergies. I knew these problems were there, but I thought they were 'normal' problems that everyone had. I never realized they were caused by foods. These food allergies might have shortened my life and the arthritis they caused may have twisted and disfigured me. What if I were one of those people that could not or would not change my diet? There are people just like I describe, who think that "What you don't know won't hurt you!"

Some of my uncles still have a very painful arthritis in their upper back and they don't know what causes it. They live with it. What else can I say? I know people that have some of the problems I mention who take medications, see doctors, and go to the grave without dying from them.

Some things, such as the arthritis in my back, did get painful sometimes, but I worked around it. I also had a lot of general stiffness in my neck, shoulders, elbows, hands, and hips, but then who doesn't over the age of thirty? It came on so slowly I hardly noticed it except maybe to think that I needed stretching and much more exercise. I thought it was 'normal' to not be able to move in the morning.

I never really felt my hair falling out or gave a second thought to my sensitive skin or even the developing wrinkles in my skin. I never thought that dozing off behind the wheel of a car or sleep disturbances were a food problem either. There were dozens, if not hundreds, of things I hardly noticed that were related to diet. I soon found out that my whole life, everything from dreams to ear wax and 'ring around the collar', was affected by what I ate.

On a more serious note, at thirty I was getting a stoop in my upper back, but then my Grandfather and all my mother's brothers had this stoop or related arthritis in the upper back. My mother's father, his mother and his mother's mother had this upper back stoop! I would be safe to say that I inherited this allergic expression from them.

I had adapted behaviorally to this arthritis. Working at counter top, such as doing dishes, or at workbench level, standing reading, or typing in an ordinary position would bring on excruciating pain. I wisely tried not to do movements or get into positions that brought on this excruciating pain. Depending upon my actions and diet this pain, which started just below my right shoulder, would sometimes block the movement of my right arm.

To overcome this problem when typing I went through more than thirty table and chair combinations. Eventually I salvaged a low seated Boston rocker, fitted it with seat and lumbar pillows, and built a typing table to my specifications to sit in a position that would not bring on this painful condition.

I visited an orthopedic surgeon who manipulated my back in a chiropractic manner twice a week for well over a year to relieve the pain from this food problem. I personally know four other people who have this type of arthritis, have been to doctors for braces to straighten up the back, and/or endured long hours of spinal manipulation and, like the members of my family, have never even thought that their problem was food related. One said that he had a terrific pain in his back from drinking beer barley), as I did. He had thought about and 'discovered' that it was a food problem also, although he didn't understand that it was related to ecology.

I went to the medical profession for other food caused problems such as headaches, asthma, and swelling glands, one of which was surgically removed. Not one of them suspected a food problem simply because not one had studied why the problems were caused by food. They all wanted to treat these food problems the way they had been medically trained 'by the book' to do, instead of removing the offending food from the diet, which may have been simpler in the first place.

Doctors now have not got time to study food problems unless it is a specialty. The problem is that virtually everyone has or will have food problems. If only a few doctors specialize, then there are a lot of doctors who don't 'see' food problems. Everyone should learn human dietary ecology and the food problems that come from it before they get out of high school! Doctors should thoroughly learn about the subject in pre med courses college health courses before they ever start to med school.

What I am saying here is that many food problem specialists who deal with food problems think that far more than half the patients who walk into a doctor's office have a food problem. But few, if any, are considering the ancestral diet of the individuals they are advising.

The main concern, even with the medical profession, is that by failing to consider individual dietary needs, an extremely few can understand the full implications of food problems. The biggest advance in medicine will not come from technology, but will come when the medical profession learns that humans are a product of evolution. Medicine must be based on human ecology for the next generation. But ecology involves much more than just food.

Chapter 7

ENERGY AND SLEEP PROBLEMS

After I discovered the basics of a diet matched to the ecology of one's ancestors I tried to match it as best as I could, given the supermarkets of today's world. After all, I would be eating these foods for the rest of my life. After I ate this diet for long periods I started noticing things I had not noticed on single food testing.

There were a lot of little things to learn. Many plant foods such as grains are related botanically. The protein complexes of these foods are similar. If you are adapted to a common descendent of a food there is a good chance that you will not be allergic to foods with similar protein groups. In other words I have no problems with sunflower seeds. The sunflower is generally recognized as North American food and I could not find mention of it as a staple in Middle Tennessee in the nineteenth century. Around the Baltic areas of Western Russia it is now a staple. Did another member of the composite family or a relative of lettuce from the Baltic area get confused with the modern American sunflower? It doesn't make that much difference, as the protein groups are similar. Cultivated foods are no different.

Animal foods also vary. I am severely allergic to trout. Trout is an inland fish and not an ocean fish. But many inland and ocean fish have common ancestors. I have no problems with either ocean or fresh water catfish. I am allergic to oysters, and also to crayfish, crawdad, shrimp or lobsters which have similar protein groups. The protein in these causes my thumbs to itch, but my digestive physiology will digest the protein, to which I am allergic.

My ancestors ate ducks and geese and now I eat chicken and turkey. There is a slight difference among these birds' protein groups. Turkeys, which are recognized as American in origin, have a chemical that gives me a headache when I eat it in quantity, but otherwise I am not allergic to it.

Of course, I went back and retested the more than three dozen foods my body was allergic to, in order to make sure that I had not missed anything or confused anything that happened with another food that I thought was 'free' of problems. This process required months to complete. In the meantime I was writing everything I noticed down, but very often I would discover things that I had not noticed.

I had noticed years ago while on a vegetarian diet that my brain felt 'slow.' It took me too long to really get my brain 'in gear' in the morning and I'll admit that my vegetarian diet days often included a lot of caffeinated tea. I have actually heard several people describe some vegetarians as 'slow brains.'

My thought processes also felt extremely slow at times. This was especially true in mid to late afternoon, to the point of taking a nap. I simply could not sit down and put my brain to task at these times while on a straight vegetarian diet. I had to keep a high level of physical activity to keep my brain working. This was not necessarily good for college studying. I used this afternoon period to play volleyball, shop, or whatever.

Studies had shown that a high protein diet for breakfast was needed for optimum brain performance. The 'transport' of 'sleep' protein is blocked by a high protein diet. I was not getting quality protein to keep from going to sleep. When I learned this I added eggs and milk back into my vegetarian diet for an ovo-lacto vegetarian diet. That worked much better, especially when I had two eggs for breakfast and a skimmed milk yogurt product for lunch when studying for college classes. But a vegetarian diet was too much trouble to keep up during college and I got back on to a 'regular' college diet, which did just about as good if not better in some ways.

For practical purposes, my food allergies make confetti out of everything I had learned from books on vegetarianism. Up until about twenty years ago, when modern medicine stepped in, the vegetarian diet was the best diet to be had for someone over forty years of age who didn't have diabetes. (Can one imagine the ignorance of a vegetarian diabetic diet book! Yes there is one.) One of the few reasons left to be a vegetarian now is for moral reasons or to make some kind of statement.

You will lose weight, and lower your cholesterol if you sincerely practice a strict vegetarian diet without eggs or milk. A vegetarian diet with defatted eggs and skimmed milk will also help heart disease and lower weight. From the time of Leonardo da Vinci, a vegetarian diet was thought to 'cure' heart disease, among other problems. Da Vinci realized he had such problems and became a practicing vegetarian! It was the only known cure for heart disease in the mid Nineteenth century, according to several of the medical texts I have.

However, a vegetarian diet does not work for everyone. One woman I know with blond hair, blue eyes, fair skin and very obviously severe food allergies and intolerances is practicing a vegetarian diet. It is pitiful to see her with severe acne and arthritis. I noticed she has many similar problems to what I once had, but much worse.

What about toxins and aflatoxins on a vegetarian diet? People of the Danube area eat corn and beans with a fungus on them that creates a powerful aflatoxin which destroys kidney tissue in those people. Bruce Ames has shown these powerful vegetable aflatoxins are carcinogenic. In other words if you are not adapted to these toxins you may get cancer from them.

In summer school I started having tuna sandwiches for an early brunch. My study performance and brain power increased substantially. I remember this quite well.

I had two servings of tea a day at this time because coffee gave me a 'jolt' or a short peak. I had to have more and more coffee to keep these peaks level. At one time I was drinking as much as six to ten servings a day and on some days as much as twenty! Coffee was my first 'food problem', as I started having stomach pains from it, not to mention the 'jitters.' The sharp jolts and stomach pain are still with me today when I have coffee very often.

When I first thought about adding protein I had not tested eggs, so I used canned 'sardines' for breakfast, because of the bone calcium in them. These are any kind of small fish canned all over the world and there are possibly a hundred different species involved. There was a good possibility that I would eat fish that my body was allergic to.

In the intervening years since I first started this dietary idea I have had virtually no problem with any kind of commercial ocean fish except tuna and some of the tropical species that are not commercial fish. Tuna sometimes gives me extremely severe headaches from the coral reef toxins it has collected in its fat. Tuna from the more northerly seas does not give me problems. Coral reefs, of course, are in the tropics and many latitudes from Scandinavia.

I started testing combinations of protein. When I ate fish three times a day my 'brain power' felt like it was double that of the days I ate chicken or turkey. If I ate turkey two or three times a day I got headaches from a known chemical in it. It sometimes disturbed my sleep. Turkey worked as well as chicken otherwise. Turkey is a North American bird.

After a few days of eating only fish protein along with five servings of vegetables in my diet group a day, my sleep period decreased to a mere five to five and a half hours. Without caffeine my sleep became extremely sound. It was so sound that at times it scared me, because I would not wake when there was a crashing storm!

I would close my eyes at night and seconds before I woke up in the morning my brain was at full thinking capacity, ready to go. There was no morning grogginess. It did not take a shower or caffeine or a couple of hours to get the 'cobwebs' out of the nights sleep. I could concentrate on extremely complex problems ten seconds after I woke up. I used this time quite effectively to solve problems or think through ideas associated with this diet.

I tried eating fish three times a day and timing caffeine and simple carbohydrate consumption with 'jet lag', and it almost negated any side effects. I almost have to do this in the spring when Daylight Savings Time takes effect. It works better than anything else when I absolutely have to function.

My brain, when eating three servings of fish a day, would function at a high capacity all day long, even through the slow middle afternoon period. I wish a thousand times over that I had known this in school, especially around exam time! When I was in college, I slept through dozens of classes and afternoon labs when I was only able to schedule them during my slow midafternoon time period. But there was a lot more to come.

As I said before it was nine months before I tested red meats. I was not ready for the first test. During vacations and in eating with others I would 'eat, drink, and be merry' and just generally forget about my diet, 'pigging out' on whatever food I liked. It was like this when I visited my parents. The trip seemed a refreshing break from our routine.

Dad had a fresh venison kill for us. We had venison steaks and venison hash for breakfast almost the entire time we were there. Everything seemed well until I started driving the two hundred seventy-five miles home. As usual, we slept in and got a ten am start. We stopped for lunch at one thirty pm, since I was feeling a little tired. Most of the time, just before lunch, I know I am hungry when I start yawning. The fish sandwich lunch didn't help the tired feeling. I realized that I had had a couple of servings of tea before we got off from my parent's house. I had a Coke and refill, which I never do for lunch. At this time I had not had any caffeine for more than nine months, and yet I had already had four servings!

Suddenly, I realized that I was driving with 'one eye open' literally, and I had just banged my head into the steering wheel! If I didn't close one eye when this happened, I would start getting double vision. My head would start wobbling from just not being awake. Sharon was asleep and I just could not keep my brain to the task of driving. I fought with every idea I could to keep awake, including turning the air vents to my face with the air conditioning on full. I had another coke and just managed to drive through the Atlanta traffic.

"I wonder if I can keep my brain to task for another hour home", I thought at this point.

What had happened to my brain? It didn't happen when I drove up to my parents and hadn't happened since I started this diet. However, I had been totally off of red meat for months. The only food that could have caused this was the venison. I have heard other people talk about red meat putting them to sleep, but I had never really tried it on myself.

I tested beef two weeks later. Starting Sunday noon I started eating two servings of beef a day, with eggs and fish on alternating days for breakfast. Anybody could happen to have hamburgers for lunch and steak, meat loaf, meat balls and spaghetti or beef stir fry for four days in a row and never think much about it.

I started having these little 'blip outs' that are described by doctors who study narcoleptics. Tuesday I woke up groggy and just couldn't get going. It was difficult to get my brain going that morning no matter how hard I tried. That same day, after trying to write at my computer, I started having serious eye coordination problems and dyslexia problems, which I hadn't even noticed before at all. After only twenty minutes of reading, the lines seemed to twist at the ends of sentences. This had happened thousands of times when I was in school and I really never paid attention to it! In school I simply took a break or stopped working or reading often for the day.

I stopped writing for the day, and started working on my car, but I just couldn't seem to break out of a slow brain mood. I had some tea, which helped, as I still was not having caffeine daily.

Bedtime came an hour earlier than usual that night and was very groggy when I awoke. I took a shower to wake up at lunch. Just thirty minutes later I absolutely had to have some tea. Less than ten minutes after I finished the tea I went to sleep for two whole hours!

I tested beef eating three times. The results were always the same. The more red meat I ate the more difficulty I had keeping awake, the groggier I was, and the more I would just fall asleep at the wrong time.

At a point before I was tired enough to sleep I would develop coordination and dyslexic problems. Quite often it wasn't a point, but more like a long twilight period. I would often have long 'blinks.' I felt like I was sleep walking in some ways.

My neck muscles would lose coordination and my head would wobble while I was driving. If this period was long enough, my vision changed so that it seemed as if I was in a tunnel. If the tunnel got blank or dark to the point where my vision was like a small TV screen at a distance I would be functionally asleep. This happened about a half dozen times while I was driving and I knew to wake up! My face hit the steering wheel only twice in 200,000 miles of driving. Luckily, both times I was on a long straight stretch on the Interstate! Could it have been that the long monotonous road was more of an enticement sleep at the wrong time?

Needless to say, I virtually never eat red meat now when I know I have to stay alert. Amazingly, I had lived with this problem all my life, thought it was normal and thought that this problem of being tired and falling asleep at inconvenient times happened to everyone. If I do not eat red meat, I do not have this problem. I have no problem at all if I eat mostly fish protein before and during a long drive.

Physical activity made my response to red meat almost unnoticeable. It only happened when I was reading, driving or engaging in other activity that required sitting still while using my brain.

Back in the late '50s it was called 'highway hypnosis.' The Interstate Highway System was designed with a curve every three miles to keep people awake! These curves were where I almost ran off the road when I got tired! Sharon appears not to have this problem. If anything, she has the opposite response, staying more alert on red meat. A woman who had been narcoleptic, as diagnosed by a physician, appeared on the Phil Donahue show describing exactly the same problems as I had, although she hadn't tested the effects of various diets on her problem. She had even started sleeping through college classes in the afternoon just as I had. I tried to never have classes scheduled in the afternoon for this reason.

About this time I noticed these 'blipouts' in other people. One girl who smoked heavily would take out a cigarette just after one of these blips. I talked to her about quitting. 'Yes' she had tried dozens of times, but… She was dependent on the nicotine to stay awake! How many marginal narcoleptics smoke tobacco to stay functionally alert?

This problem with daytime sleepiness was compounded with simple carbohydrates. The more carbohydrates I had the worse the problem of sleeping during the day became. I realized this even in school. If I had more than two tablespoons of honey in my tea, sugar, or waffles and pancakes with syrup for breakfast and/or lunch I had afternoon problems, unless I had a high level of physical activity. Caffeine tended to 'burn off' this carbohydrate load somewhat if I did not have red meat. But the effects of caffeine did not completely wear off.

Quite often I would have periods in the afternoon where I was in an 'in between' situation. I would not be tired enough to sleep, but yet I would have the dyslexic brain twisting. I saw the dyslexic specialist Dr. Harold Levinson and got some helpful information, although I could not stay on any of the drugs which he prescribed for prolonged periods. Several foods affected my dyslexia. Basically, I was born with an inherited defect in that my eyes would not operate together. Eventually, with work, they became less problematic, but I still had a learning disability from it. I got through college working around narcolepsy, dyslexia and eye problems!

Caffeine added to this dyslexic problem. It caused what I would call 'skip errors' and 'brain overrun' especially if I had too much. My brain would not think in straight linear ways, but with caffeine it would more often skip or overrun ideas to the point of skipping words or flipping letters or numbers. Basically, on caffeine my brain worked faster than it could structure the things I thought about. To learn to type with fewer mistakes I had to get off caffeine. With a computer I can type out a piece and not worry too much about mistakes.

This dietary shift from a local dietary ecology to a global agriculture dietary ecology has produced many problems and adaptations to those problems, such as a cup of coffee, intense noise stimulation such as in loud music or driving loud cars, tobacco smoking, and even in scheduling classes!

Do people actually smoke as way to a stimulate them to wake up from a narcoleptic situation caused by eating the wrong foods? These people may be some of the ones who can't quit. Smoking cuts down ones sensitivity to stimuli such as food allergies. Once I could 'see' what allergies and narcolepsy were like, I first noticed them in smokers! No wonder people have a hard time quitting smoking.

Chapter 8

ARTHRITIS: THE DISEASE OF A THOUSAND CAUSES

There are well over a 100 recognized causes of arthritis, including poor nutrition, age, venereal disease, Lymes' disease, and dozens of parasites. No one can do justice to the subject just by making a few statements.

I make no claims for anyone else! I will explain exactly what I know and have learned about food caused arthritic problems in myself and how I got rid of the pain of arthritis just by changing my diet. That is all I can do. If this works for anyone else, that would be great, but it may not! No one will have exactly the same set of foods that work for them as I do, because their ancestry, the genes they inherited and the foods that their ancestors were exposed to will not be the same. Only a few members of my family will be similar.

I know dozens of people, like a vegetarian mentioned earlier, who have joint pain caused by food allergy who are terribly confused about the part food plays in arthritis. I view arthritis as an ecological problem. Ecological thinking may help solve some of the worse arthritic problems.

Until I started on the 'allergy find', diet I never realized arthritis could be caused by foods. After reading accounts' dating back to the 1950's and earlier about how some doctors had 'discovered' arthritis was caused by food allergy problems, I was stunned. When I first discovered I had food induced arthritis the idea that food could cause joint pain was not widely accepted in the medical profession.

In my early 20's, after a long motorcycle ride or a long day driving anything, my neck and sometimes my hands would be stiff. I would sometimes have to try with great effort to remove them from the grasping position of the steering. Other parts of my body would be stiff. It sometimes took several hours of loosening up to feel normal. At this point, some of my joints that got stiff would 'pop' for a relief effect.

A few years later I went to an orthopedic surgeon who was skilled at manipulating joints. I felt good for about twenty-four to forty-eight hours after he treated me, but then I needed this manipulation done again. Office visits were limited to twice a week, but sometimes I could have gone every day. I kept this up for over year. It offered only temporary relief and nothing more. Note that I went to a physician about this problem. He did not know of any long-term solutions to my pain

It was interesting that my upper back would get stiffer during the day into the evening, which wasn't at all like morning stiffness. Unlike 'brain' tired I felt a 'lack of energy' tired in my upper back and muscles, but I still felt intellectually competent. I just didn't want to move. I just wanted to relax about the dishes that needed to be washed. Doing the dishes brought on the most gruelingly painful condition I have known. This tired 'lack of energy' and this extreme pain from working at counter top conditions was the first stage in what I now know was a grain/fruit pectin/gum allergy.

Gradually, at first unnoticed I started losing range of movement in my elbows, neck, and shoulders. Almost unnoticed also was a stiffness in the morning, particularly in my neck and shoulders. These joints also were the most painful when I was sick or had a fever. I didn't realize that this last part could be vitally important in understanding this type of arthritis or even rheumatoid disease.

I hadn't been on my new diet for long before I found I had four different arthritic areas that were caused by different families of foods. Pseudo-gout had been slowly enlarging the largest joint of the big toe on my left foot. It took a long time to become problematic, but one morning after a party I awoke to pain. I had eaten four foods that cause an attack at once. I had pickled herring, oatmeal cookies, and some wine along with a cola that afternoon. After that I was careful, but when I had black-eyed peas, vinegar chicken, and a beer at a party it came back. At this point, it took a combination of several problem foods. The herring and chicken were both soaked in vinegar. An added cola put too much acid into my system. I had no problem with ordinary chicken or herring. Add alcohol to either vinegar recipe and one food, such as oatmeal or beans, and you have a mix for gout. It doesn't take much to figure it out when I have charts right in front of me.

This was years before I started the allergy diet, but notice how vinegar, oatmeal, beans and cola, where not part of my ancestral diet. Note that beans and grains make up a perfect match in the vegetarian diet. It becomes easy to notice these things when someone points them out. I rarely have problems with gout now unless I drink colas. I inherited pseudo gout from my mother's mother.

When I started this diet I was shocked that I found that grains caused me arthritis and intense pain in the region of my 3-4 thoracic vertebrae. I had been duped by the 'goodness of whole grains' idea. It is ironic that I am allergic to the very thing in oats that is supposed to lower ones cholesterol. The soluble fiber which has been the subject of so much news because of its effect on reducing cholesterol was the problem. This arthritis also included many of the high pectin fruits, especially jams, jellies and preserves with added pectin. Cellulose gum and some other 'gums' also cause this arthritis. These are used in a variety of foods, such as most syrups, and as thickening agents in sauces.

About six months before I started this dietary venture, I tried to straighten the 'stoop' that had been developing in my upper back from my mid 20's. Every time my mother saw me she would say, "Straighten up your shoulders or you'll be like your uncle". She was referring to one of my uncles had a back brace when the stoop in his back developed in his late 20's. Eventually every single one of my uncles developed this problem to some extent, except one uncle who smoked heavily. My mother's father died with a stiff 'C' shape in his back. He had reached the point that he couldn't lie flat on his back on the floor. His head would not touch the floor when he tried to.

My uncles and I would have severe pain just under the left or right shoulder blade. Sometimes this pain or stiffness was so bad that it would extend down to the hand on either side in numbing pain. Some of their X-rays showed bone 'spurs' in the 3-4 thoracic region of the back. My X-rays of this region showed very little of anything that would cause a problem, but the pain was unmistakable. (X-rays were taken when I saw yet another doctor about this problem.) These were not the high resolution studies that can be taken of a joint today, so it's impossible to say what was there in the early stages of development.

I could not lie flat on the floor on my back for more than a minute without pain, but I could still touch my head to the floor at this time. After six months of trying through physical exercise, but before beginning my allergy diet, I had made a little progress in straightening my back against the floor. Then, after a few weeks totally off all foods that affected the area, I was able to lie comfortably and straight on the floor.

It took me another six months and I could sleep for hours on my back without pain. At this time I had also regained most of the movement in my neck and back. It felt wonderful. I had previously lost at least forty percent of the side to side head movement range from eating foods such as whole grain oats. As I loosened up I regained the ability to glance over my shoulder. Most of the pain was gone within a week after I was off all foods that caused the arthritis, but it took six months off of all foods with which I had problems before I fully regained the flexibility of my youth. Thus, we are not talking about a quick fix that can be accomplished in a few days. It can take a lot of time and effort to return a joint to normal. In my case, I caught the problem relatively early, before the severe joint damage that had happened in my uncles was present. However, if a person does not find the diet that is appropriate for them before the joint is severely damaged, it will not be able to rebuild itself.

I found these foods one at a time over several years of testing. All grains except wheat and corn gave me noticeable problems. I seem to have a 'partial' adaptation to wheat and corn, which my more recent ancestors ate. Barley, buckwheat, oats, rice, and rye all cause me excruciating joint pain, as well as the high pectin fruits such as apples, pears, and dates. Other foods such as sweet potatoes, cranberries, and many forms of 'soluble fiber' or gum are also included. Technically not a food, MSG or monosodium glutamate also contributes heavily to the problem.

One of my worst problems is barley. I cannot eat any bread anywhere unless it is Middle East style or Kosher. If you start reading labels, you will notice that almost all commercial breads, cereals, cookies and crackers have added barley, barley malt, or a variation thereof on the label, and worse yet some have barley in them but aren't labeled as such. This list, of course, includes beer and brewer's yeast. Anyone can well understand how and why I needed to find a set of foods I was not allergic to.

There is another set of foods and spices that give me arthritis in my hands, hips, and lower back! Lower back problems are a leading cause of days out of work in this country! My lower back problem is mostly caused by one family of foods called the 'night shades', and by many spices. These include tomatoes, potatoes, eggplant, and all kinds of peppers from green and red to chili, paprika and tobacco. Then there was ginger, cloves, and other pickling spices, which also gave me stiffness in my hands.

One other food causes me an arthritic problem, but it is not like the others. While sleeping on my sides, my shoulders get sore only when I have a lot of milk or acid type foods such as orange juice. The project of sorting out all these foods would have been almost impossible without writing everything down and knowing that there was a set of foods that were clear and free from all symptoms, including joint pain.

I still eat some of these foods on occasion and if they cause me a problem I simply take ibuprofen or aspirin as a 'morning after' pill. The worst foods or spices, which often give me arthritic stiffness or pain all out of proportion to the amount I eat are barley, concentrated pectins, MSG, ginger, cloves, and paprika.

Even years after I discovered the foods that cause me arthritis, I keep finding something that I have missed. Usually, it is in a factory made food or recipe. For instance, I was having syrup on French toast. I started getting stiffness in my upper back from this. I found that the syrup was thickened with 'cellulose gum.' This gum or soluble fiber caused me arthritis. Plain honey or pure corn syrup did not cause my arthritic stiffening problem with the same bread and egg combination. Another time it was 'cottonseed fiber', which was obvious. I had to use my brain on this.

Then I discovered the injury type of arthritis! How many more can there be? One day I stepped on a stick in the driveway and fell backward onto the two middle fingers of my right hand. These fingers were bent over backward at the first knuckle. Over the weeks these joints hurt and kept hurting. I had to drop the small amount of spices and night shades I had allowed into my diet for two months until these joints 'healed.' In other words these foods kept these joints, and no other joints, sore.

This brings up the question, "Do these foods accelerate the normal 'wear and tear' type of arthritis?" Obviously they do. Without extensive knowledge of foods I would have just had 'normal' arthritis, treated by 'normal' doctors who had no idea that foods can be a contributing factor in arthritis! Without a base of foods that caused me no problems whatsoever, I would not have been able to find these foods, one by one over, a period of years!

You have to READ LABELS, READ LABELS, AND READ LABELS to avoid food stocks that have added ingredients that may cause you problems. I have found over thirty-six foods, spices, and additives that cause me joint pain and stiffness, and the number keeps growing. It is not simple as taking a pill and the pain is gone. It is a constant vigil to keep these foods, spices, and additives from destroying my joints, but I have the knowledge to do it. It is not easy.

One hundred percent of the foods that cause me arthritic problems are not native or indigenous to northern Europe, especially the islands and shores of the eastern Baltic Sea where my father's paternal ancestors came from.

Several other things caused me arthritis. I had an arthritis that I couldn't find a food for. It kept getting a little worse for about a month. Then my infant son was bothered by pin worms. In such cases, it is usual to treat the entire family. Three days after taking pin worm medication the arthritic pain eased up and never returned again. The entire time I had been eating foods that cause me absolutely no arthritic problems.

One Friday started off great. I had eaten foods clear of problems since the Wednesday before, but I felt off. It wasn't really the time of day to be tired and so I just kept struggling along getting things done, but I felt that I was having a severely allergic response to something. However, I hadn't eaten trout or any other food that was a major problem.

Sharon came back a little early and thought I looked flushed. She put the inside of her wrist on my forehead and immediately said that I had a fever! I had never realized it. Historically, my joints felt achy when I had fever. I then realized that my joints were not aching because I was not eating the foods that caused them to ache. I had always had joint pain when I had a fever, but I wasn't eating foods that caused aches in my joints so I did not have aches and did not realize I had a fever.

Several years later, I started developing painful joints and immediately I got off all foods that caused me any arthritic problems, and started eating nothing but my core diet. It did not go away. I noticed I had a minor sore throat for several weeks before. My tonsils and glands in my neck were slightly swollen at this time. It was reported that some cases of rheumatoid arthritis have been alleviated by antibiotics. I went to a GP and told him about my swollen glands but not about my suspecting arthritis. His strep test was negative. To be on the safe side he gave me a prescription. I took the antibiotic and within forty-eight hours my minor sore throat and arthritic condition subsided. I don't normally take antibiotics and am very leery of over prescription.

When I get a fever causing microbe while eating any of the foods mentioned above I get extremely painful joints. If I have a fever and I am not eating any of these foods I have no pain. It appears that joint pain is a multifaceted situation with many complexities. Without knowledge of basic ecology I would not be able to control my arthritis. It is not a simple situation. I have to live in this culture full of foods that cause me problems. There are sixty million people in this country who have arthritis. How many millions of people who have arthritis from routinely eating foods not eaten and adapted to by their ancestors is not known. If even a tenth of them are affected by foods the way I am, that would be six million people! That is a lot of people. We need base line studies of what percentage of the population are affected by food induced arthritis!

It all started because the 'goodness' of whole grains caused a stiffness in my upper back and neck. All of this stiffness and pain in my joints was happening in my 30's. If I had not discovered this and still been eating these foods in my 50's and 60's, would this have contributed to the so called 'wear and tear' type of arthritis? I can't make recommendations

for anyone in this case, but I would suggest
that anyone would be much better off eating a
diet very close to what they are adapted to.

Chapter 9

VISUAL VANITIES

Once I had discovered the foods that appeared to match my physiology, they comprised at least seventy-five percent of my diet. After about six months, I started noticing little changes that I hadn't been particularly paying attention to. These things were subtle and at first I couldn't relate them to specific foods, but this eventually changed.

I started losing significant amounts of weight. I really didn't need to lose weight, as I was already slim, but at the end of six months, I was down to what I had weighed as a junior in high school. I took a significant look into this diet and found that it was naturally low in fat, with a much higher vegetable content than I'd been eating before. Without butter fat, fat from red meats, added oils such as soy, corn, or cottonseed, my diet at this time had far less than half of the fat of the average American diet. I didn't even think about counting calories.

Most people think fat (or oil) is fat and that is that. But each individual's physiology handles different fats and oils in different ways. I know people who can eat all the fatty foods they want and stay thin like me and people who can eat all the saturated fat they want without undue health problems.

Years ago when I finished my degree in college I noticed in the pictures that were taken at that time that my hair was becoming very thin. I went to my ten high school class reunion and was voted one of the three who had lost the most hair! I now have three times the hair. My beard was thin in areas on my cheeks and other areas where I had had acne. These areas started growing hair with this diet. My mustache and beard hair grew larger in diameter, longer and denser at the same time. When I looked closely, hair had started thickening and growing in places I had never had hair! After nine months on this diet, I was growing hair in places that had previously only grown fuzz. This was particularly nice for my scalp.

In a freshman biology class we had examined our thumbs for hair. The teacher mentioned that some people have hair on their thumb, and it was a recessive genetic trait. I had none. When I looked at this time, 5 hairs were growing on my right thumb. My left thumb had nothing but scar tissue in that area. But then, hair was growing profusely on all my other fingers and toes and my hands, my arms, my legs, my body and yes even on the top of my head. My eyebrows had errant hair that was growing out thicker and more profusely than the other hair in my brows. Where there was fuzz on my head before there was hair!

I mentioned this in conversation several times and typically received a response of incredulity. "You're pretty strange really telling a tale like this," one friend said. I realized that I had exceeded the level of credibility. Who would believe that there was a diet that will regrow hair? Doctors only have chemicals for that, like minoxidyl.

For about two weeks I retested milk, which a skin prick test assured the doctor I was allergic to. This retest was to make sure I actually had symptoms. Did I have symptoms! After nine days on milk products, I noticed while brushing my hair that the brush was getting full of loose hair. My pillow was coated with a mat of hair that was steadily falling out. Cessation of consumption of milk products ended this.

I realized with this that any situation may be caused by a multiplicity of factors. Like several other conditions such as arthritis, if you have more than one food causing problems then you can get very confused. Toss in several other factors such as injury, poor nutrition, etc. and you better know how each factor affects the situation.

After I'd been on my new allergy free diet for awhile, I noticed that my wrinkles were not as deep on my face, especially around my eyes. However, at times I would have deep wrinkles and 'bags' under my eyes. These bags corresponded roughly with my eating red meat and/or especially beef fat! If I ate a lot of beef fat, the 'delicate' skin around my eyes would puff up and 'bag.' I tried this more than half a dozen times with just beef fat. Again and again and again this happened. There wasn't any question that beef fat 'aged' me ten years!

Again, I told some friends this and they were disbelieving. Really, would you believe someone making these claims about a diet? I found references to exactly what I experienced in a book dated in the 1920's! Someone else had observed this fact also.

If I knew the exact physiology of this process, I would explain it here. The book from 1925 explains that the heavy fat plugs up tiny blood vessels around the eyes. The fish may have a better balance of protein, collagen, and fat that my body is adapted to. With my thin blood from a low cholesterol diet, these areas get more nutrients.

Long before I started all this, I had noticed that when I ate a heavy fat meal I often got a 'greasy queasy' feeling in my gut. Some other oils and fats, such as cottonseed oil, actually make my gut hurt when I eat more than a small serving of potato chips fried in this oil. The feeling is like a large lump in my gut. I can eat an entire bag of potato chips fried in sunflower oil without this pain. Cottonseed oil has just crept into the backdoor, as cheap oil, since the 50's. I know my ancestors didn't eat large amounts of beef fat and didn't eat cottonseed oil at all. I try not to buy any food with cottonseed on the label. I have not explored all the effects of these oils, but some do have an off taste or after taste. Cottonseed does affect my taste.

I had discontinued shaving many years before due to chronic problems with shaving rash which the various doctors I had been to had been unable to resolve. Once I had been on my allergen free diet for several months, I started shaving, after a ten year hiatus, and there was no shaving rash. For the first time in ten years my skin wasn't all that sensitive. Because of digestive problems with cheap substitute fats and oils and the beef problem, I started testing each oil and fat separately, just as if each was a separate food. I then tested some real butter and there were no stomach problems. However, instantly, with the next shave the rash came back. This didn't exactly fit the allergy pattern, but at the time I didn't think about it.

Later I discovered that it involved an etiology that has never had scientific scrutiny. It was in testing each oil and fat separately that I struck another dietary gold mine, but it would take me a while to figure it out.

Peanut butter and peanut oil gave me severely painful adult acne pimples. I had not had pimples this painful in years. Three other very specific things caused me adult acne. They were Mozzarella and Romano cheeses, a particular brand of soda, and soy products. Peanuts and soy are botanically related and not native to Scandinavia. These Italian cheeses were not cultured in Scandinavia either and of course I am allergic to milk. What do I not have to say about the complex mess of artificial ingredients in soda?

I avoided all soy products for a year, as well as the other specific oils that caused me problems. In the meantime my skin cleared of all blemishes, redness, and scar tissue related to acne. I couldn't remember a time in my life when I had been without these red blemishes. Then I started eating soy oil products again without problems. This was puzzling.

Note here that some leading acne specialists have concluded that intake of fats has nothing to do with acne. Again, if you have more than one element causing a problem, then it becomes difficult, if not impossible, to sort these out without an organized plan. Human ecology can provide the basis for an organized plan. If you generally cut total fat consumption and one or two particular fats still in your diet cause acne, then you will miss the point. In my case, only specific fats and oils cause acne. I had to single them out one by one, just as if they were food allergies. Generalizations such as the idea that fats do, or do not, cause acne are not useful. Someone else might be tolerant of peanut oil, to which I have a severe response, and intolerant of fish oils, which I can consume without any problems.

Chapter 10

A STRANGE ETIOLOGY THAT HAS HAD LITTLE RESEARCH

I kept running into the idea that certain specific foods act as a medium, sponsor, or otherwise cause certain specific bacterial pathogens to grow. These specific foods and/or pathogens are not native or indigenous to the ancestral home of a particular individual.

After having not eaten red meat for nine months, I started eating beef twice a day for three days. Suddenly, I noticed that my clothes had an extremely intense odor. This was particularly true of my socks. Why did I lose this odor or not have it when I ate fish and chicken?

I once experimented by not taking a bath for two whole weeks in the summer while I was totally off red meat, milk products and eggs. At times I did very sweaty work, but I just changed clothes every day. My wife didn't even notice and thought I had taken a bath over lunch or whenever she was not there. She notices once I add eggs back to my diet.

When I was seventeen I dropped a 152 lb. paving form on my right little toe and smashed the nail. Before the toe nail healed a fungal infection set in which I had for fifteen years. The toe nail grew back but was soft and flaky. Eight months after I started this diet it was growing back more or less normally and I didn't have the fungus! Years before a dermatologist had told me that I would have to have the toenail surgically removed and the infection treated. I never had the time to see about it, but the diet I was on had cleared it up and this was unmistakable. There are diets that supposedly cure fungus and yeast problems, but again the ecological approach may work much better.

In athlete's foot, the attending bacteria can be as much of the problem as the fungus. It was after my toenail got better that I thought about how the eating of beef caused the intense smell of my socks and clothes. Everybody knows that bacteria are the cause of this intense body odor and the usual solution is to simply take a bath and use deodorant. Research has shown that the most rapid growth of these bacteria is immediately after a shower! Even the most intense scrubbing with an antibacterial scrub will not get into the deep recesses of the nails. Wouldn't it be more effective to shut off food to these bacteria? If the immune system is at strength and the bacteria are 'starved' out of existence at the same time, the infection may be 'cured.' What does this mean for other infections? In other words, does the food that feeds body odor bacteria cause other bacterial problems?

Three hundred years ago bathing wasn't very common. Back in those days people were eating closer to their natural ecology, because there were no trains and trailer trucks to haul food around. It was during the Renaissance that soap began to be produced in quantities, and when people of lesser means were able to eat larger quantities of novel foods.

I had noticed this intense odor once before, as a vegetarian going back to the 'normal' American diet. I talked to several vegetarians about this and found that many of them had experienced this intense odor when eating meat for a while when they visited the home of their parents or restarted eating red meat for convenience.

I found a number of foods that caused bacteria to grow profusely on my skin and cause a smell. You may have guessed it. These foods were mostly red meat animals. When I ate fish, chicken, and frogs odor causing bacteria did not grow as swiftly. All red meat fats that I tried, milk fats, and eggs caused these bacteria to grow in profusion. The longer I was off these foods the slower it was for the smell to come back. I tested them over and over.

Basically, what you have in these animal foods is nutrients such as fats that are a surplus of food which human bodies are not adapted to use. What happens to this surplus? It is consumed by smaller organisms just as in any ecological situation. Scientists think that a diet with heavy fats such as these grow bacteria in the gut which produce toxins. These toxins are thought to irritate the cells that line the gut, causing cancer.

These organisms may cause dozens, if not hundreds, of disease problems not thought out and described by the medical community. One was a shaving rash which I had for more than ten years. I remember specifically that this rash started when I was at the University of

Tennessee. It ceased when I stopped eating milk fats.

Some, such as the organisms that cause baby colic (which are described later) are a severe nuisance if not the cause of much child abuse. Others like acne hideously scar teenagers' faces for life.

Acne is caused by a pathogen that can often be controlled with antibiotics and other bacterial control agents. It also can sometimes be controlled with diet, especially subtracting the generalized 'greasy' foods. The question is can bacteria be specific? Lactobacillus is specific.

The adult acne bacterium that causes me problems appears to be very specific. In other words, there are specific foods that result in the growth of pathogens and these foods follow a specific ecological order. The big problem with many of these organisms is that every member of the family, and everything the affected person touches has to be free of the organisms that cause the problem or the person can be reinoculated again and again, even if antibiotics and medications are used to treat them.

The fats in these foods that I have found to foster bacteria growth so far seem that they could be a complex of fats and protein in some cases. Lipofuscin or a combination of fat and protein could be the culprit. In other words these bacteria are food specific. Quit eating the food and the bacteria perish.

Then the thought occurred to me. What if a person were allergic to one or more of these organisms? Acne appears to be such a disease, but are there others? There are many reasons to believe such an allergy exists. You eat a food, say milk, and it grows a bacterium which you are allergic to. Your immune system would build a titer from the constant presentation, but you would never show an allergy specifically to milk.

Interestingly, there have been a number of antecedents dating from the nineteenth century, declaring that when removal of the animal foods of red meat, milk, and eggs from the diet alleviates some or most of the suffering of rheumatoid arthritis. Interestingly, also, fish, chicken, and turkey do not seem to affect rheumatoid disease. Some American medical texts of the Nineteenth Century prescribed a total vegetarian (vegan or no meat, milk or egg) diet for relief of rheumatoid disease. This idea has been largely ignored because many plant foods can also contribute to, arthritis such as potatoes and tomatoes. Milk and milk products were the foods that caused me night sweats, which some doctors think is bacterial in origin.

Some scientists think rheumatoid arthritis is caused by a transmittable pathogen or pathogens, because it shows up in Native Americans before the time of Columbus. There is no description of it in Europe before the sixteenth century. It has many of the symptoms of a pathogenic infection, including low grade fever and increased immune responses. Some cases of rheumatoid disease have responded to antibiotics. If it responds to antibiotics, there is a good chance some forms are bacterial. Being chronically presented as it is, it could develop a resistance to antibiotics. Bacteria are sensitive to iron. It may also respond to a lowered iron intake.

Remember that eating certain vegetable foods caused me simple allergic arthritis. My joints had even more pain from these foods when I acquired a pathogen that caused a fever. In other words, the immune system is excited by any pathogen and simple food allergies are turned into fierce joint destroying agents. As with other pathogens, a person can be continually reinoculated from his or her environment. What an incredibly complex etiology. Are there specific foods that sponsor the growth of specific organisms that may be pathogenic?

Having witnessed such an occurrence, I would say yes.

You will note that pathogens, like foods and humans, have spread worldwide. Some people have adapted to some pathogens. It is simple ecology, really, although the complexities could number into the millions. It is time to use computers to sort out these problems. Dietary scientists must start thinking of many diseases in terms of human dietary ecology. We must have individual evolution added to dietary studies.

Chapter 11

LEARNING TO MANIPULATE FOODS: BABY COLIC, INFANT ALLERGIES, EAR INFECTIONS, TOXINS, TEMPER TANTRUMS AND NIGHT TERRORS

Human dietary evolution may be used to solve all kinds of problems not now thought to be related to food. For some of these problems, the medical profession does not even believe there is a cure, or else they deny that the problem is really a problem.

The 'three month baby colic' is widespread and yet the medical profession basically says "grin and bear it"! I know because I've been there. I wish I had known at the time that we could have affected a cure by following simple ecological principles. As I experimented with this dietary experience I began to realize how important this idea was. Most of the medical profession does not even have an idea of what food problems are like and why they exist. They also don't realize the scope of food problems.

I read a lot of scientific literature written about the subject of food and quite often I read grass roots or popular literature often dismissed by scientists. In every single incident thought to be connected to food, few individuals used evolutionary or ecological thought processes to solve food problems. Usually, generalized nutrition or generalized ideas based upon a single dietary idea, such as "Vitamin C is good for you", was used to try to explain what were really dynamic ecological situations. Results with this approach may be limited success or dismal failure. Many food problems are a combination of actions or a dynamic situation where any number of things could affect the problem. A new field of study called something like Medical Dietary Ecology needs to be created.

Our son, from the day after we brought him home from the hospital started having problems with severe colic. He was in constant distress, crying and screaming night and day. I was ready to do something, anything to end it. It was stressful on Sharon and me, but the constant crying was a clear indication that our son was in distress. Slowly I got used to it, but I hated every minute of it. Our pediatrician could really offer no suggestions. Simethicone and vibration or rocking was the well established treatment at the time our son was born. It did very little good and whenever we would call the doctors to report that he was still crying, we were just told to give more simethicone, rock him, and wait for it to end. From every indication, I learned it was a food problem, but how could it be controlled?

When Sharon was pregnant, she had been consuming four times the amount of milk and ice cream as she had been before she was pregnant. There was a lot of literature promoting the benefits of calcium in milk products. I knew from my moderate allergy to it that it could cause problems

Our son's entire diet consisted of his mother's milk, but still he had intensely severe infant colic. If colic was a food problem, then the mother's milk had to be part of his problem. Milk is made from what the mother eats. Even though Sharon was having no allergies or other clinical problems with cow's milk, our son possibly was.

By the time three months and three days had passed the colic had passed, but my interest in it had not. I noticed several things, including baby's body odor. He sometimes smelled like cheese. Was there a culture acting upon the milk in his gut? Basically, there are thousands of organisms that grow on milk sugars, fats, and protein. From the first mammal millions of years ago, lower organisms feasted upon their milk. Humans have learned to deliberately 'spoil' milk in the making of yogurt, cheese, or other cultures to keep even more harmful organisms from poisoning it for human consumption. But we ignore some organisms, such as the ones that cause skin odor or grow in our gut with milk consumption. It is the organisms of this 'ecology' that causes a baby so much discomfort from colic.

Before delivery, Sharon had been consuming massive amounts of milk products. Various organisms may have utilized the parts of the milk that she could or did not utilize. I believe that these organisms which depend upon milk for survival could have been 'starved out' if she had gotten completely off milk products for as little as one month before our son was born.

In preparation for our next child, Sharon totally discontinued use of milk products a month before her due date. The child had almost no colic. This 'fasting' from milk and milk products was just enough to break the culture of organisms related to milk consumption. Our pediatrician said she had heard that avoiding cow milk products before birth may affect colic in some individuals, but she did not know the specifics!

We also ate very little red meat during Sharon's second pregnancy, which may have helped rid our bodies and habitats of the bacteria and other organisms that grow on milk fats, sugars and proteins, thus contributing to our second child's healthier first three months. This ecological disease, with its incessant screaming in the night is the cause of many strained relationships, child abuse and infants beaten to death to get them to stop the incessant screaming. While Sharon and I just held our son and walked him and rocked him until we were exhausted, many parents find themselves unable to cope.

After that colic period of our first born, the next four and a half weeks were pleasant baby weeks. For some reason they went extremely fast. Then it happened! Our son got cold, followed by ear infections, with screaming in the night hour after hour. We went the usual round of doctors etc., but our son kept going downhill. He developed asthma and chronic ear infections. In this time we saw seven different doctors, including specialists, who gave our son ten different medications and spent a lot of the insurance company's money, not to mention a lot of our own, and in the end he was still sick. We used antibiotics until he either became allergic to them or we knew they didn't work. We finally went to ear tubes for the chronic ear infections, but his chronic asthma and the medications he took for it were the main and immediate problem.

The allergy specialist said, "Hang in there. At least your son is stable."

I posed a question. "What if I can find the cause of his asthma and then take him off medications?" I already knew even then that the medications were a major part of his problem. I had been to the pharmacy and read the exceedingly small print giving all the indications, contraindications, problems, side effects etc. of the medications he was taking. Sleepless nights were one of sons' main problems! As a result of the stimulant effects of the medications, he was getting hardly any rest. Neither were Sharon or I. The allergist said I could not possibly find the cause of allergies, but we were desperate. I looked into the mirror and saw dark circles around my eyes.

Sharon was even worse. The skin around her eyes was not only darkened, but it was also sunken deep into her eye sockets. She had a haggard pallor like one sees in someone dying. In spite of the physicians and the medication, our son was still sick. Desperation was a great motivator to try something else.

I had spent what little free time I had researching our son's problem and had just concluded that dietary evolution could be used. I had spent more than forty hours working on the problem, reading about everything we put into our son's mouth. I checked all the pharmacological contraindications and side effects on all of his medications as well as every vitamin and mineral or other element in his formula. I even looked up the possibility of the rubber nipples or some element such as sulfur in them causing him problems. Everything from the water and soap used to wash and boil the nipples and bottles, to the distilled water we used with the formula came under suspicion. We had two wonderful Manx cats that we gave away at this time because the doctor recommended it.

Rule #1 in identifying food allergies. SIMPLIFY THE DIET.

The fewer different things you put into your mouth, the easier it is to find a food problem. Indeed, I used mostly the rules of the latest clinical allergy thinking, with my own twist. There were too many elements going into his mouth.

There were at least a dozen ingredients in his baby formula. According to my ideas of ecology, it was relevant that none of the ingredients of the formula and none of the medications we fed him were indigenous to the area of his ancestors or had been eaten by them. At least one of these elements, I was certain, was the cause of the asthma. If we used ONE FOOD, in his case one milk, then we could build from there, but it could not be cow's milk.

I also had suspicions that the vitamins and simple iron in his infant formula might be 'feeding' his ear infections. At the time, he was on a soy formula in hopes that that might help. I had deliberately picked the low iron formula. The soy and safflower oil, as well as the carriers of the manufactured vitamins, were not in ancients diets.

Raw soy is toxic to humans. Could soy be suppressing his immune system? Could the protein in soy be inadequate in forming the white cells and other proteins needed by the immune system? Toxins can and do often suppress the immune system, but what was important? The most important point was that soy was not eaten by Scandinavians.

The most dramatic diet would be to feed him a blenderized version of my diet, with some of the solids removed if he had problems with all milks. Like father like son. If immune unresponsiveness is inherited paternally then it would be a bonus in this case. As Sharon was blonde and blue eyed this might be close to what her ancestry ate also.

We could try a milk that was common to Scandinavia, such as reindeer milk or goat milk. I was allergic to cow milk, so I ruled it out. The choice was simple because reindeer milk was scarce in Georgia, where we were living at the time. Goat milk was readily available from local goat dairies. It was a single food and we could tell immediately if he was allergic to it. We could also easily tell if he was developing an allergy to it. My doubts about goat milk were few, but there were always more drastic diets.

My idea was simplification and change. There was virtually a one hundred percent chance that if his allergic problem was a food, we could find it. When there was only one food to deal with that was near what our ancestors might have consumed as opposed to a multiplicity of things our ancestors never consumed, the likelihood that goat's milk would present the exact same problem was extremely small.

At the pharmacy and in the Physicians' Desk Reference I had already learned about his medications. One was chemically similar to the caffeine and theobromine found in coffee and tea and the 'side effects' were often sleepless nights. In other words, it was as if he was on about six cups of coffee day and night. He was 'wired'. If one of the elements in the infant formula was giving him the problem, then we could take him off the medications and he would sleep like a normal baby.

Through the readings I was continuing at this time, I discovered that coffee and tobacco were both used in the nineteenth century for relief of asthma symptoms. Teddy Roosevelt smoked as a child to quell asthma symptoms. But I did not want to quell the symptoms; I wanted to find what caused them!

There was also the chance that soy was challenging his immune system. The allergist noted that his immune system was at the bottom end of average of immune output.

"For some reason his immune system just isn't putting out," the doctor said.

The vitamins and iron were, I thought, 'feeding' these infectious bacteria and his immune system was not responding well to them. If the nutrition in his formula was so good, why didn't his immune system respond better to these pathogens? I had little doubt my idea would work, but would it help his ear infections and asthma?

OK, I was guessing! But it was a well educated guess based upon sound ecological and evolutionary principles and everything I could read on the subject. If he became allergic to goat's milk as a consequence of regular exposure to it, it would take at least a couple of weeks, six at the outside. If nothing else it would buy time for us. Even this much time would give us some much needed rest and get us out of the dead of winter. The date was the twelfth of February. From my allergy knowledge and experience I was sure that the change would work.

We discussed the idea with the pediatrician, who knew all too well everything our son had been through. She was diplomatic. "Goat milk is low in folic acid and several other elements including iron, but babies around the world are raised on it." When the doctor said 'low in iron' I jumped at the idea.

Luckily, because Sharon is a veterinary professor at a major university she found a ready source of goat's milk and we started our son on it the next evening. To say that it worked is an understatement. The results were spectacular. It worked swifter and far and away better than even I had expected. It took less than twenty-four hours for our son to breathe easier. Totally off medication in thirty-six hours, his sleep problems (and ours) disappeared. He did wake once in the middle of the night, hungry, but that was easily solved and nothing compared to the six to ten times he had been waking up in distress night, after night, after night, after night. The medications that caused him the sleep problems ended! The endless doctor visits decreased to a normal level. Eventually, the ear infections cleared up.

After less than one week off the stimulant medications but breathing easily, he slept through the night! Within four days Sharon's pallor had vanished and I felt more alert and rested than I had since it began.

The next step was to find out what else he could safely consume. I took the ingredients listed on the last formula can and started adding them to the goat milk, one single element each week. I started them on Friday and later on Thursday, because if they caused problems, we would have the weekend to deal with them. I added plain soy, safflower oil, etc. The vitamins presented a problem in that I couldn't be sure they were the same as in the formula, but as our cabinet was full of individual vitamins I could see if any one of them caused him problems. Nothing! None of the single vitamins caused a problem.

Then I took half of one of Sharon's prescription maternal vitamins and ground it up into the goat milk. He had a minor case of wheezing! He quit wheezing after that one dose. I could have tried the vitamin tablet three times, but it would have proved little as it was a multivitamin. He could have been sensitized in utero! But which part of this multivitamin was causing the problem?

I started on the single minerals. The very first mineral I tried, chelated zinc, caused immediate and full blown asthma. There had been chelated minerals in his baby formula and in the maternal vitamins. I had fed them to our son 'back to back'. In other words, the first one reactivated his allergy and the second one hit full blown, as described in the allergy texts. A trip to the doctors and another course of prednisone, combined with total avoidance of the chelated zinc in any form, brought him back to health.

In the meantime, I was taking the maternal vitamins and became asthmatic. I took the same chelated zinc and had an immediate full blown asthmatic reaction! Both were obviously similar. Like son, like father.

We had spent thousands of dollars on doctors and drugs, and our son had suffered terribly, for an allergy to a simple mineral binder. I had in practice defined how to find food allergies in infants.

I still had my doubts about goat's milk, but a problem showed up seventeen and a half months (nearly a year and a half) after we started our son on goat milk. Our son was doing quite well, and then there came a violent storm. The weather had been absolutely dry for six months and then suddenly, on a ninety-six degree day, it began to cloud over and rain. At first it seemed like an ordinary thunderstorm. Then there was a very cold wind at least thirty degrees below the heat of the day and, within seconds, it suddenly turned into a ninety mile per hour microburst, ripping limbs from trees and bending those that did not break over to the ground. It was one of those severe down draft wind shears that trash airplanes.

Sharon grabbed our son, hurried away from the windows and doors and covered him. That night he had an unnerving, screaming night terror. These continued over several nights and then eight days later he had a violent temper tantrum. The minor fussiness he had before seemed like nothing compared to this.

Over the next two weeks the temper tantrums continued and became longer and more frequent. Several things disturbed me. He would be watching his favorite taped cartoon movies, like the Care Bears, and become extremely fearful of characters he had viewed many times before and never had a reaction to. Certain shapes caused him to become fearful when the lights were dimmed and he became anxious and very 'clingy' when he was dropped off at day care.

By far the worst problem was he that became fearful of me after I woke him from one of these night terrors. His fears became worse over the weeks. The temper tantrums got worse. He would go blindly thrashing mad for twenty minutes. Before these started I could talk to him out of a bad mood, but not anymore.

Both grandmothers dismissed this simply as the "way it is" when kids get "out of sorts".' Some of the books I had read on food problems in kids emphasized behavior problems. Some of the medical community expressed the need for comprehensive food testing as a cause of such diverse problems as behavior changes, which led me to the conclusion that our son probably had a food problem.

These problems corresponded roughly with the 'witching hour' and 'low blood sugar' times. I noted every single factor of these blind temper tantrums. All but one occurred between 3:40 and 5:20 pm and the violent night terrors roughly occurred between 1:15 and 3:50 am. Why these time periods?

I suspected toxins for several different reasons. The goat's milk was the main suspect, as cow's milk gave me sleep problems, headaches and sometimes out of control dreams. Milk could have several kinds of toxins.

I had worked with a toxicologist at the USDA station when Sharon was studying for her veterinary degree at the Auburn Veterinary School. Some of the plants seemed extremely toxic and caused several problems in animals. It seemed possible that they could cause behavior problems in humans. This was not like allergies, as it was sometimes random. In other words, the intensity of these problems varied. Random problems seem hard to find, but I returned to my habit or writing everything down to the last detail.

"The goat's milk is his problem," I told Sharon.

"How do you know? I thought you put him on it because it was the best thing and now (seventeen months and two weeks later) you say to take him off it."

"I just know it is the milk. Look, from the start I didn't think goat milk would last six weeks. Just be glad it lasted this long!"

We took him off goat's milk and that solved most of his fears, night terrors and temper tantrums. He still had bad moments, but they were more in keeping with a normal toddler's bad moments.

I ate the remaining goat's milk in the form of yogurt. As with every food that affects our son, I also try it. Goat's milk, unlike cow's milk, didn't cause me too many physical problems, but I noticed that I had strange and fearful dreams at times when I had it after dinner. These dreams were random, but often the themes would be similar, such as I was climbing a castle wall or a tile roof where tiles or bricks would fall or break off in my hand. At times during the day I would have strange and sometimes fearful thoughts. Driving long distances I would often be scared the car would break.

I talked to our supplier of goat's milk. She took extreme precautions to keep the milk from bacterial contamination and the toxins that went with contamination. We tried various versions, such as fresh, canned, and powdered goat's milk and I noted that our son reacted differently to each. The temperature at which they were processed seemed to make a difference. I read that many toxins break down with higher temperatures. But these milks also came from different locations, such as north Georgia, Arkansas, and California.

One thing I noticed was Kudzu and hundreds of thousands of mushrooms growing on the farm where the fresh goat's milk was obtained. The owner explained that the reason they got the farm cheaply was because the Kudzu had taken over. The mushrooms had appeared after a violent storm raked the area, the same storm that happened the day these problems began, and the rains had returned. She had had to supplement the goat's diet with hay and grain during the previous dry spell to keep up milk production. She said the goats loved the mushrooms that sprouted after the long drought ended. Could some of these mushrooms be toxic and the toxins come through the milk? Could moldy hay, silage, or even a fungus that grew on spring grasses pass toxins to cows or goats, and would these be passed through the milk? Even though the cows and goats are of European descent, the plants and lower organisms that they eat may be of North American descent.

I learned that the horses which started my quest had aborted fetuses for about three weeks during the spring when a fungus that produced a potent aflatoxin grew on the grasses here at the University of Georgia. This is where I wish I knew much more about toxicology and the way toxins affect people. I went to the library and read up on all the latest scientific accounts of toxins and milk. Some molds that infest milk do produce toxins.

I also found that undigested protein complexes from the food that the mother eats could indeed be in milk, but I couldn't find evidence of whole toxins being transferred other than that some scientists had found pesticides and heavy metals in milk. The amount that affected me and our son must have been very small, but the mental consequences could be catastrophic. I couldn't prove that toxins were actually the problem without extremely expensive tests. No one had seemed to have done an index of how toxins affected human behavior, as Doris Rapp had done with allergies and intolerances.

I could write a book on just the questions I could ask about toxins. But why were the symptoms confined to what parents call the 'witching hour' and why did night terrors occur in the specific time limits I noted?

A lucky break came slowly along. Gradually, we realized that our son had temper tantrums and night terrors from other foods. For several reasons, these did not appear to be allergies.

For one thing, they were irregular. If he ate large quantities of corn chips or popcorn in the evening, he more often than not had night terrors. One night he ate a six and one quarter ounce can of tuna and had a night terror. If he had a morning peanut butter snack at nursery school he had afternoon temper tantrums.

I tested these foods myself and found no real problems at first, although on rare occasions I got severe headaches from eating too much tuna, but this also happened with turkey, which didn't seem to affect our son.

Then I ran across a list of 'natural' food toxins by Bruce Ames of California who noted that these natural toxins are more carcinogenic than pesticides. My entire list of foods causing serious night terrors and temper tantrums were also on Ames natural toxin list! Corn and peanuts grew fungi which produced a virulent aflatoxin. Tuna was at the top of a chain of smaller fish and concentrated coral reef toxins. But just as important, all of the foods on my list of foods that were causing him problems were not indigenous to our Scandinavian ancestry, and therefore these toxins could not have been adapted to.

Native Peruvians have little or no reaction to green potato skins or eyes. European women still abort fetuses on occasion from these parts of the potato that contain a potent toxin. The potato is native to Peru. Coral reefs are about as far as one can get from the fish the Scandinavians ate. Suddenly, I realized this diet may be far more important as a scientific 'tool' than I had at first imagined.

One of the aspects of toxicity in foods is that it can vary tremendously in any given sample. Accordingly, the body may metabolize these toxins up to a point. What comes out is an on again/off again reaction that may never be correlated with the specific food. The only way to recognize toxin problems is to know specific individual adaptation to a toxin.

Most of the medical texts and books on rearing children say that violent, aggressive temper tantrums and night terrors are part of childhood and parents should just wait until children 'outgrow them.' This period lasts from about two years (eighteen months by some accounts) to eight years. Our son did 'outgrow' this period immediately when dietary toxins were eliminated, just as he would have 'outgrown' the need for infant formula and the life threatening asthma caused by the mineral binder it. I still wonder about the abnormal fears and childhood mental problems that could have shaped his personality. Do toxins affect people's personality more than anyone realizes?

For more than four decades food has been written up as the cause of mental problems. In this period there has been debate and disbelief in the psychiatric community and yet there has not been a guideline or baseline in the manipulation of foods to prove that food could be a major factor in any mental problem.

Everyone believes that 'bad chemistry' exists in the brain of disturbed individuals. As food is nothing more than complex chemistry, why hasn't the scientific community fully realized that foods could cause at least a sizeable amount of mental problems?

One psychiatrist in New York in the early '70's discovered that taking his patients off all caffeine before he saw them got patients problems to levels manageable by the patient most of the time. Otherwise, his patients just needed someone who would listen to them. In a small percentage of patients this did not help their problems. These patients needed real psychiatric help. Sigmund Freud, in the midst of the nineteenth century coffee capital of the world, didn't even notice that caffeine often disturbed sleep and accentuated dream sleep. Had Freud discovered that caffeine caused increased anxiety and exacerbation of fear in some of his patients the psychiatric world would be looking into food as the cause of mental problems such

as,depression,manic-depression, and schizophrenia!

After we had identified all the foods that caused our son problems, either due to allergies or toxins, he remained in perfect health for nearly four years without so much as a cold. When our second child was born, we used all the knowledge we had gained in raising our first when selecting her diet. She was a much healthier baby and toddler.

130

Chapter 12

MORE LEARNING TO MANIPULATE FOODS: MORNING SICKNESS

Native Peruvian women, living where the potato was first domesticated, are not likely to abort fetuses when consuming the green skin and growing eyes of potatoes. European women, on the other hand, are still likely to abort fetuses when consuming these toxins. It is not surprising that adaptation has to be at every level and aspect for a complete adaptation to a food.

Food toxins that come naturally from foods or the bacteria and fungus that grow on them can create subtle problems. One symptom appears to be the very discomforting morning sickness during pregnancy. Early in her second pregnancy, Sharon had a lot of morning sickness, worse than in her first pregnancy. Sometimes she couldn't eat anything all day. Although morning sickness is thought to be caused by high levels of pregnancy hormones, especially progesterone, other factors can be at play.

The descriptions of morning sickness and the fact that the mother's system is absorbing toxins from the fetus could also be a factor. The actual symptoms led me to believe that morning sickness was the result of excessive toxins. I reasoned that if the mother ate foods with toxins not indigenous to her ancestry then she might have the problems of morning sickness.

Sharon stopped eating the foods on the toxin list, including milk products and her morning sickness abated immediately. Although it did not completely go away, the symptoms were reduced to tolerable levels! She later told me the she sneaked milk products without problems a few weeks later!

Could toxins from bacterial action on milk in the gut also cause this? In other words, when she quit most foods except milk, the organisms in her gut that were feasting on the milk died out. When she had milk the next time these organisms were not there in numbers to cause problems.

One of the interesting sidelines is that thalidomide, which caused deformities in babies, was used to treat this morning sickness into the 60's. What other problems can eating a diet not adapted to cause?

Chapter 13

WHO HAS ALLERGIES?

In reviewing the scientific literature on diet I was amazed at the sheer mass of work that could be challenged, dispelled, or dispatched by using ecology or evolutionary guidelines. In this era of science, using generalized nutritional studies as a basis for diet is absurd. It isn't really a wonder that modern medicine is confused about diet. When evolutionary adaptation to food is used in human research we will have a much better understanding of how an individual needs to go about designing their diet. Evolution is a fact of life. The physiology of a person is adapted to a set of foods found in a limited ecological area. Along comes this global agricultural dietary ecology and we have unrecognized food problems. This change in diet was a fact before the 'scientific rules' and observation methods were in place. I estimate that, using the current medical descriptions, definitions, and 'proof positive' tests of food allergies about seventy-five percent of the people who actually have food allergies aren't counted. There is no baseline on which to do research on numbers. How can we know what is and what is not a food allergy, intolerance, or even a problem if we do not use an ecological adaptation baseline?

It is hard to imagine an area in science today that has no baseline. FREE BASING DRUG IDEAS ON MEDICAL PROBLEMS WHICH ARE ACTUALLY FOOD ALLERGIES OR INTOLERANCES INVITES DISASTER, but that is what we are doing. Many FOOD PROBLEMS such as mine are tossed into a 'nondescript' immune or autoimmune problem file, or I am told that I don't have a problem! "We now have excellent medications that will cover your allergy problems."

Using evolution and ecology for dietary problems will increase the numbers of people who have food problems to virtually all of the population! Some will have extremely minor problems that may never be noticeable, while others will have more problems with more severe reactions. For instance, someone may not call 'morning stiffness' caused by milk toxins or peanut aflatoxin a problem, but it could be worse. Saying that someone who currently has minor symptoms doesn't have food allergies is like saying that someone who has HIV does not have a disease.

We should teach evolutionary dietary factors in high school health classes. (Note that when I talk evolution here I mean since 4004 B.C. In other words, this has nothing to do with monkeys!) Certainly, by college everyone should know this as basic science. All pre medical courses should include evolutionary adaptation to diet.

With our better understanding of human evolution we may find dietary factors that started 40,000 years ago. It may be something like Eskimos that are not allergic to elephant meat because they ate mastodon or we may find a way to save endangered wildlife. Certainly, I have stated how delicate and balanced ecology can be.

Chapter 14

THE IMPOSSIBLE TASK

A friend listening to my ideas said, "All this is wonderful, but do you realize how impossible it is. IT IS ONE THING FOR YOU TO FIND THIS OUT, BUT TO PUT IT INTO PRACTICAL APPLICATION IS IMPOSSIBLE. There are thousands of factors and hundreds of foods to consider and you just walk in and tell everyone how easy it is. I realize that a friend of mine who has a Greek name, a Greek nose, and four Greek grandparents is going to have a relatively easy time, while another friend of mine who has an Irish-Apache father and a French-Vietnamese mother is going to be more problematic. But you don't say it is impossible to everybody, because someone will always be there to prove you wrong!

Even I have a somewhat mixed ancestry. There are Scottish, Irish, Welsh, English, French, Spanish, German, Prussian, and Scandinavian names in my ancestry. From my explorations of my food allergies and foods without immune reactions, I have only one ancestry that could have contributed to my immune heritage.

Chapter 15

IRON-THE DOUBLE EDGED SWORD

I can still remember when scientists first proposed that the body used fever during sickness as a way to deny the mineral iron to bacteria. Indeed, I had noticed that my son's ear infections decreased substantially when we fed him low iron goat milk.

I noticed that I could eat an iron fortified food after dinner and even with brushing my teeth, I would have a rotten mouth the next morning. I deliberately ate foods low in iron and breads with no added iron and the bacteria in my mouth subsided! What damage do iron fortified grain products cause to teeth? If bacteria cause tooth decay, what if we reduced the iron available to these bacteria

With kids in preschool, I caught all kinds of bacteria and viruses until I tried stopping all extra iron and went strictly to unfortified foods. When everyone in the family got strep throat, I didn't come down with it. Once, when they had a bacterial problem, I ate a bunch of iron fortified foods and immediately caught their infection.

Having cleared my son's chronic ear infections on a low iron diet I now firmly believe that we could reduce many if not most of the prescriptions for antibiotics. We could reduce complications from pneumonia and infections and inflammation in general.

The dentist said I had gingivitis at about the time I quit eating all iron fortified foods and used salt to brush my teeth. That subsequently cleared it up! In the simple iron fortified breads iron may be in a form that pathogens have evolved to utilize faster than the human body can.

One more area where iron is damaging could be with cardiovascular problems. As a person ages, the body generally has higher stores of iron. It has been found that the more iron stores a person has after a heart attack the more 'damage' is done. Antioxidants are needed to help prevent this damage.

Incredibly, even with little or no red meat and no 'reduced' iron on this dietary regimen I have more 'energy.' The one thing I have not done is check to see how my iron levels have varied. The doctor's clinic where I have a full physical every year has not mentioned that I have a low iron level.

If iron fortified foods do indeed affect pathogen problems in humans it would cause a major upheaval in food 'manufacture.' If many ear infections could be cleared up by putting the patient on a low iron or natural iron diet it would revolutionize medicine and food.

Chapter 16

AUTOIMMUNE AND OTHER PROBLEMS

One of the allergists I talked with mentioned how far insight into the immune system has come. In the 1950s before food allergies had really been explored, virtually all arthritis except for some caused by venereal disease was thought to be 'autoimmune.' THE BODY ATTACKS ITSELF. It was like autoimmune was a catch all file that everything got classed (thrown) into.

Many allergists, such as Doris Rapp MD, have books with long lists of which specific foods cause which specific problems most often, but it seems that none of these fine allergists explore the native ecology of the individual. Many, like Theodor Randolf MD, have, since the

1930's, insisted that more people have environmental food, airborne, toxin or whatever intolerances, but still don't take the necessary step over into true ecology.

When ecology is used we get a very clear picture of what allergies are and exactly why they exist. IF WE USE THE ECOLOGICAL VIEW OF THE HUMAN DIET, THEN VIRTUALLY ONE HUNDRED PERCENT OF THE POPULATION AT ONE TIME OR ANOTHER WILL EXPERIENCE A FOOD ALLERGY OR INTOLERANCE PROBLEM. Whether they or their doctor know it as an allergy or intolerance depends upon a multiplicity of factors.

For instance, milk causes my blood vessels to swell, possibly from histamine release. When I eat foods not native to Scandinavia that have specific toxins or proteins I often get severe headaches. One summer when I was in college I drank a lot of milk and hot chocolate and lived in a dorm room with newly installed, out-gassing carpet and enamel paint. I was in the clinic at least a dozen times for severe headache. I SAW A MEDICAL DOCTOR FOR THIS PROBLEM!!! At this time, also long before this diet started, I would buy a pound of M&Ms or a stack of milk chocolate bars and 'pig out.' The next day I would have severe headaches. I could eat chocolate without milk or milk without chocolate and not have these fierce headaches. I quit eating chocolate for nearly ten years.

Now it is known that specific foods cause arthritis and more than a hundred other causes have been discovered. I discovered that subtracting certain foods and spices from my diet relieved most of my arthritic symptoms within a week. As I explained before, not one of these foods, such as chocolate is native to the ecology of Scandinavia where my ancestors lived. How much arthritis is caused by what people eat? We will never know until baseline studies are done using the principles of human dietary ecology.

What if, in eating this diet, a person still had arthritis? In Rheumatoid arthritis the immune system actually attacks the body's cartilage or connective tissue, independent of these specific foods. Medical books from the middle of the nineteenth century suggest that arthritic inflammation decreases if red meats, milk and eggs are deleted from the diet. They don't say to eat fish and chicken exclusively. Why didn't anyone follow this up in modern medicine?

One day I read through some old <u>Scientific American</u>. In one issue I read that the immune system can distinguish down to the molecular level, even to the point of different molecular structure. Then I read that the French wine industry was cracking down on wine makers for using cane sugar as opposed to grape sugar in their wines. This was made possible by modern technology that can distinguish the molecular difference between these two sugars. Why does lactobacillus languish in cane sugar, but multiplies rapidly in lactose or milk sugar?

It is obvious with food allergies that the immune system can distinguish between all sorts of proteins, lipids, and polysaccharides and that pieces and parts of larger molecules are found in the bloodstream.

It is a fact that larger pieces of 'foreign' protein can get into the blood stream. The digestive physiology does not digest everything totally, as we assume, especially 'foreign' food protein. Could the body use these different bits of protein for building blocks just as they are? Could the body use amino acid strings, lipids and other larger food particles that are 'foreign' to build itself before the immune system learns to respond to these specific built in food particles?

The human body can utilize insulin from cows if injected, but the digestive process will break most of it up if ingested. For that matter, the body can use all sorts of hormones and enzymes not made by the human body. Many human proteins are similar to most mammals. Notice I use the word similar. They may work, but are they a perfect match? Will the body use these for building blocks?

Perhaps as an individual keeps eating this specific food protein, the immune system becomes ever more aggressive toward these food bits USED IN BUILDING THE BODY, which it recognizes as foreign. These specific food structures are built into the body structure and, ZAP, the system then starts attacking this part of the body.

An example would be a person whose ancestors had lived near the Baltic coast eating Baltic estuary and sea creatures for as much as four or five millennia and then suddenly the person's family moves to American heartland. In America the person starts eating venison, beef, and pork. A cosmetic surgeon injects 'purified' beef collagen to fill out a persons wrinkles. Suddenly the body starts attacking itself.

For scientists sake let's not be over simplistic. There are dozens if not hundreds of pathogenic organisms that can commandeer the body's cells to do their bidding while the immune system tries to destroy them. In the best way it can, the body is programmed to kill the pathogen or the cell host.

IF WE DON'T KNOW THE FULL EXTENT OF FOOD ALLERGIES HOW CAN MEDICAL SCIENCE ESTABLISH A BASELINE FOR 'AUTOIMMUNE' DISEASE?

One major theory of aging is that the DNA makes replication mistakes. How would this dietary protein shift humanity has undergone affect this replication mistakes? Could this dietary shift cause a lot of them? <u>FOOD ALLERGIES ALONE CAN DO A LOT OF TISSUE DAMAGE</u>.

Basically, in the overall scheme of life, all this does not amount to much, as the evolutionary rule applies here. Life is programmed to continue itself through sexual reproduction and a few individuals who have minor allergies or autoimmune problems are just part of the mix. If they reproduce they pass on their genetic codes with a few modifications.

Chapter 17

FASTING

Fasting has been practiced since ancient times for either religious purposes or to conserve food stores. Fasting was also used in the ancient world to cleanse the body of 'toxins.' Ancient peoples were forced into total fasting when food stores ran out at various times because of drought, famine, or a long winter. It is no coincidence that Lent, or religious fasting comes at the end of winter or just before the new crops come in.

One reason nutritionists do not like total fasting is that the water soluble vitamins are almost totally gone in forty-eight hours. It is dangerous to do this for longer periods of time.

Nothing is wasted when the body is in this fasting mode, as virtually every part of the body interacts to secure nutrients from the available food or from the body itself for vital functioning. This is just one reason, when fasting for longer periods, to use medical supervision.

It is interesting that ancient peoples went months at a time without specific vitamins. A study of many peoples three hundred years ago would bring up the question of, if fasting is that bad, why could these peoples survive at all? Studies of humans today indicate that many people of means have incredibly poor diets. Indeed, many people on 'junk food' may actually go for years with diets low in some nutrients, and yet they manage to function. When studying ecology I learned that all living things need nutrients. If denied specific nutrients long enough they die out, or markedly slow reproduction.

About three years before this diet started I drank milk fortified with a malted vitamin and mineral enrichment product. After a few days of using it I got an incredible flatulence and gas. The lactose, iron, and B vitamins made a perfect nutrient rich environment for lactobacilli to wildly reproduce, causing me these gassing problems. I discovered that these lactobacilli would die out if I had little or no lactose!!! This also happened when I had a certain brand of cereal that had 100% of the RDA of iron.

Somehow about this time I realized I was becoming lactose intolerant. In other words, my body did not make enough of the enzyme lactase to digest all of the milk sugars, but it was much worse when I had 'reduced' iron supplements along with the lactose. It was simple enough to eat cheeses and yogurt, but these products kept many forms of the lactobacillus alive. Little did I know that I would truly be allergic to cow milk in less than three years.

Little did I know then that there were numerous foods besides milk that caused bacteria to proliferate in and on my body? In other words, the nutrients that my body did not use or could not use fast enough provided a perfect ecology for these bacteria to reproduce, often excessively.

Incredibly, I was allergic to some of these bacteria or their byproducts, but not the specific food. When I got off the foods that caused the growth of these pathogens, I starved them by changing their ecology. I could find little, if any, mention of controlling pathogenic bacteria by fasting. Little did I realize then how extensive these pathogens that grow with the consumption of specific foods are.

These pathogenic organisms were noticed in the mid 19th century, especially with the consumption of animal products. Medical doctors noticed that people on a vegetarian diet had less inflammation. Why or how could they notice this? A red meat diet provides a higher intake of iron and, you can guess, a faster growth of bacteria.

As far back as the fourteenth century, it was recognized that heavy meat eaters had a heavy body odor. Many vegetarians have told me that going from red meat in the diet to a plain vegetarian diet and back again to meat eating, they notice a decrease and then an increase in body odor. We now know that bacteria cause most of these odors.

In some people, heavy meat eating causes these bacteria to proliferate, probably from the hemiron in the red meat. Can these bacteria cause inflammation, as the nineteenth century texts describe? Can people actually be allergic to these bacteria? What if it was an inflammation like rheumatoid arthritis? It has been reported in some journals that people fasting have reported a reduction in rheumatoid pain and inflammation! It has been reported that the animal foods milk, eggs, and red meat have been shown to exacerbate rheumatoid problems.

Could this be true? There have been several antecedents that say it can.

The main thought I have about this is that the rheumatoid pathogen needs nutrients, and even if a person doesn't eat red meats, milk, and eggs the body may have enough stored nutrients for this pathogen to cause problems for six months or more. Most people want results quickly or a 'quick fix' by the medical profession. We have gotten used to instantaneous results, but dietary results can take much longer.

The growth and spread of organisms connected to specific foods may be attributed to continuous eating of red meats, milk and eggs. In the ancient days these foods were not available constantly day after day. In other words, we can have eggs seven days a week for years if we want them whereas the ancients never had eggs for more than a few days in a row.

Many creatures, including ancient humans, seem to have adapted to this feast or famine situation in the wild, while in modern developed countries it is always feast for most humans. Between famine and the bodies natural defenses, many bacteria including some pathogens may be controlled or die out completely in the wild.

Few people realize that fasting can have medical uses. Medically, fasting is used in clinical allergy to start finding allergies and intolerances. If you have food allergies, most will 'clear' with forty-eight to seventy-two hours of fasting. Some take as much as two weeks of fasting under a doctors supervision to clear.

If you started with a 'clear' set of foods in the first place there would be no need for fasting. (I suspect that some 'autoimmune reactions' may take years if not decades to subside even if a perfect diet is eaten.)

Several other actions have effects similar to fasting. In the nineteenth century 'evacuating the gut' by various means was considered a necessary medical procedure. Ipecac was given to the patients for this purpose, as were enemas. Often, heavy laxatives or toxins were given to patients for the gut to expel its contents. They didn't know why or how these things worked, and often used them for the wrong situation, but they did put pathogens on the defensive and starved them at the same time.

Just a little over a hundred years ago people believed that anything that caused a reaction was 'toxic' or poison. Toxins, in the ancient world, could be anything that the body reacted to, including food allergies or intolerances, as they were not knowledgeable as we are today about how food affects a persons physiology. There were a lot of things that were actually toxic. Ancient peoples could not understand diet the way modern science can fathom even the minutest dietary problem.

Fasting and/or eating in times of scarcity adapted humans to better absorb specific nutrients and specific protein of a particular ecology. In other words, some people who lived near the sea may have survived on an ounce of fish and small bits of seaweed and seaside vegetation for many days on end during the winter and can eat these foods without any problems whatsoever and even thrive on small amounts of them.

In a modern sense 'dieting' or trying to cut back on the amount of food one consumes is actually the closest thing most modern people come to 'fasting.' In ancient times, fasting did not necessarily mean to completely stop eating, but more often was the cutting back on the kind or the amount or adhering to a strict regimen of food and timing when the food was eaten. Such diseases as bulimia, anorexia nervosa, and overdosing of laxatives are also related to fasting, in a deliberate attempt to reduce weight. These diseases are mental, but are thought to have a physical basis.

A major reason that many people complain they are hungry or that they don't feel good eating a weight reducing diet is the elements of that diet may not be readily absorbed or utilized by their physiology. Another major reason may be that the individual may actually be allergic to the few foods they are eating on their diet. For instance, virtually all of the 'liquid diet' drinks have milk, milk protein or parts of milk in them, which a good percent of the population is allergic to or at least not adapted to. Some of these drinks have gums I am allergic to. Others have vitamin and mineral binders that I am also allergic to.

"Why fast or skip a single meal when we have plenty to eat?", was a question a relative once asked. I personally would rather eat nothing at times when I have a gastrointestinal problem, or if I have eaten a food to which my immune system profoundly reacts. I 'fast' from the foods that cause me problems!

Chapter 18

TO QUIT SMOKING

One of the things I noticed was that several members of my family started smoking later in life than was the norm of starting as teenagers. I also noticed that those who smoke don't seem to notice their allergies as much! This was especially true of one of my aunts and one of my grandfathers.

My grandfather smoked so little I never realized it until late in his life, but he started smoking more as his allergy to MSG and grains caused an ever increasing stoop in his back. My aunt hated people to even smoke around her and didn't have the habit until well into her forties! This was as her allergies started showing.

Tobacco smoke is one of the smokiest smelling smokes there is. Needless to say people that smoke smell like something that has been burned over. Certain fabrics like wool sweaters and even hair hold this smell. And smoker's breathe is terrible. A captivating beauty like even Catherine Deneuve loses some of it when she smokes.

Smoking is really a filthy habit. Not only do smokers smell bad, but they make the environment in which they smoke smell bad. Once I watched a smoker drop ashes on the produce in a major supermarket and toss the burning butt on the floor. I said something about it to the manager. He and I mentioned this to a municipality that was contemplating banning smoking. That was all it took. There is no question that smoking gives a bad flavor to the food you eat in a restaurant. It ruins the taste of good food. It gives me headaches.

There are a lot of studies dealing with tobacco now. The best medicine a doctor can recommend for tobacco users who have ulcers, headaches and heart problems is to give up smoking. Women who smoke during pregnancy are fifty percent more likely to have retarded babies. But with all the data there are still a lot of people who can't give up smoking and tobacco.

The reasoning is simple. Nicotine, the principle active chemical, is addictive. It is funny to see someone doing tobacco in one form or function and say that they despise people on drugs.

They're hooked on the best selling one yet. Nicotine is supposed to cut down on the small sensory perceptions so the person can live in this modern world without getting nervous breakdowns or whatever. But even when the modern world is taken away, many still can't quit.

Just from my observations, I get little aches and pains from food allergies. What if all these aches and pains are negated when a person uses tobacco? This was recognized in the 1840's. No wonder people can't get off tobacco. They have all these little aches and pains and other problems from the food they eat. When they stop the 'feel good' chemicals released when they are using nicotine, they feel rotten. In other words, all the little subclinical food problems become noticeable after one stops nicotine. I know that relatives have these aches and can understand why they can't get off tobacco.

And the real hitch is that tobacco is one of the notorious Nightshade plants that are proven to cause arthritis. I asked why one of my kin stopped chewing tobacco and they said that it hurt their joints! It is from the Americas.

Chapter 19

SUGGESTIONS FROM HISTORY

One of the most celebrated changes in diet observed in ancient times was that of Samson of the bible. He changed his diet from that of his humble ancestors to that of Delilah's courtiers and became weak in strength.

Observers who then did not understand this dietary change ascribed the change in his strength to the length of his hair, which was obviously the most visible manifestation of his courtly change. It was stylistically cut short when Delihla seduced him into the life of her making. Everyone should know that the length of one's hair has little if any meaning other than one's hair is long or short. If one understands ecology and can see past these red herrings there are a lot of historically recorded changes in diet that have produced problems.

Dietary change was also noticed to bring on health problems by the ancient Greeks, but they lacked the means to understand in minute detail why these problems occurred. 'Exotic' or imported foods in Greece in those days were noticed to cause reactions in some individuals. Changes in diet, especially in the more affluent people actually were a mixed bag. These changes did increase the lifespan for some individuals in this class of people, but others showed signs of problems.

The vegetarian diet, at least from the time of Leonardo daVinci, was 'observed' in the scientific fashion of the day to be the best diet for many ailments. DaVinci, who probably had weight and circulatory problems, switched to a vegetarian diet because even then there was evidence that it helped 'cure' these problems.

The growing wealth of ordinary people of the Renaissance led to a massive change in diet. This change was the beginning of 'diseases of civilization.' Scientists of the Renaissance could not observe things in minute detail as we can today, but then they also did not have in place the scientific principles of investigation.

There are hundreds if not thousands of observations of dietary change in historical references that most scientists have not really examined. Did Marco Polo have dietary problems? Tomatoes and potatoes, when first introduced into Europe were considered to be poison. Of course, in those days the reason for anaphylactic shock from the consumption of a food was unknown, but poison was poison. 'Poisoned' was a term generally ascribed in those days to any known reaction to any ingested food stuff including food allergies. The historical accounts of someone poisoned may be inaccurate. No one knows how many people actually had allergic problems with the introduction of New World foods into Europe. Only a few researchers really ever thought that these foods could cause enough allergic reactions to actually kill someone. The poison in green potato skins and eyes to this day will abort fetuses in some European women. In the eighteenth century when a woman miscarried it was just a miscarriage and no one realized there could be a connection to a food. Peel the potatoes and there is none.

For years we have actually seen historical examples and not realized that they were depictions of food problems. History is littered with instances where a change in diet causes problems. Subtle instances dating back in time are easy to read about. Henry the third's son John loved French cheeses, but had a pimpled face. Now there are indications now that milk products are a relatively major cause of acne problems.

Many people such as Theodore Roosevelt, or Sir Henry Royce of Rolls-Royce fame had food problems. Just reading their biography points out where their diet was problematic.

Often, it takes months and sometimes years for a specific food eaten regularly to give the least hint of a problem in some people. Even today, many people of European descent with 'morning stiffness' or even major arthritic problems from 40 years of eating the North and South American 'night shade' group of vegetables will simply ascribe it to growing older, not knowing these mild symptoms will subside when these foods, among others, are deleted from their diet. I, for instance, thought the same thing. Having eaten a fairly standard American diet for thirty plus years, why should I notice something that had come on slowly for the last ten years? It took several weeks to several months after I stopped eating the night shade group of foods for my hands, hips and lower back to loosen up, even though the pain or soreness stopped almost immediately.

I don't necessary like to eat these select foods. I don't have to tell anyone that I love the taste of many of the foods I can't eat. I had to take each food and find ways to prepare it so I would like it.

Chapter 21

CONCLUSION

At this moment, we are free basing ideas of human diet on nutrition without any hope of settling many dietary mysteries, such as diabetes, dietary arthritis, or even simple headaches. Many of these problems are ecological problems that go unsolved, because we don't teach students in medical school how to think about, discover, understand, and solve ecological dietary problems.

We need comprehensive studies on how dietary change has affected humans since migration changed from a very slow process requiring years and generations to a rapid process in which people are constantly moving themselves and their foods around the globe. With these studies we can better understand and define the complications of immune physiology or any disturbance of physiology caused by diet. Even now, I realize that there could be dozens of physiological problems with just one food. Clinical immunology cannot wait on this, no matter how many complications or how difficult, and we cannot go back.

From these baseline studies we can markedly improve human dietary science. We can better understand the rate and maximum change of human evolution, as food allergies and other dietary physiological disturbances are one of the most visible signs of human evolution.

We can better understand how to deal with ecological problems affecting life on earth. It doesn't take much to see that we have burned our bridges and totally changed the ecology of many areas of this planet much faster than humans have and can adapt to this change. To make matters worse, various genetically modified foods are rapidly being added to our food supply. In many areas it is already too late, but that is not to say that we don't need the information now.

We need these studies if we are to have any hope of long term space exploration. We have got to go where no man has gone before in the study of diet, simply because men have got to 'eat' in space. But this brings up another more scary aspect of space travel. Will our earth bound immune physiology, when it comes in contact with 'alien' species of any kind be totally allergic to them? Is there a human genotype that will accept most forms of life without being severely allergic to just shaking hands. Is there only one 'way' life can develop? Why do we have to know?

In the meantime, the individual reader is left with the question of what all this means to them and their health. Unless you are descended primarily or entirely from natives of Scandinavia, my answer will not be your answer. To find your own answer, you will need to find out as much as possible about who your ancestors were and where they came from, and then study their dietary traditions. Learn what foods were native to the locale they came from, and what foods were imported to the area where they lived and at what point in history. When you are ready to begin, start with a simple diet with only a few foods, or even one food, if necessary. When you are sure you have found at least one food that you are tolerant of, try gradually adding others, making reference to what your ancestors ate. Of course, before beginning such a drastic dietary change, you should discuss this with your physician.

To end with the adage 'EAT, DRINK, AND BE MERRY…' is not compatible to this book or to a long life for most people. It would be more appropriate to say a line from Star Trek. 'LIVE LONG AND PROSPER.'

About the Author

William (Bill) Crowell was born and raised in Shelbyville, Tennessee. His dietary interest began in his youth when he often ate wild game including deer, squirrels, frogs, rabbits, dove, quail, and pheasant. He earned his B.S. from the University of Tennessee in 1974. At the university he was exposed to myriad variations of diet. Afterwards, his interest in dietary problems soared when he discovered the scientific contradictions of being allergic to many highly nutritious foods. His search for the solution to food related health problems led to the discovery of important rules that are neglected or ignored in today's dietary science.